NUTRITIONAL GUIDE

A COMPREHENSIVE REFERENCE FOR BETTER HEALTH

SECOND EDITION

LOUISE TENNEY, M.H.

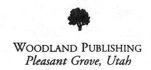

WOODLAND PUBLISHING
Pleasant Grove, Utah

© 1997
Woodland Publishing
P.O. Box 160
Pleasant Grove, UT
84062

Printed in the United States of America

NUTRITIONAL
GUIDE

A COMPREHENSIVE REFERENCE
FOR BETTER HEALTH

SECOND EDITION

TABLE OF CONTENTS

PREFACE

Men dig their graves with their own teeth and die more by those fated instruments than the weapons of their enemies.
                                        Thomas Moffett, 1600 A.D.

Many people eat without thinking about what they are doing. They are hungry, so they go to the refrigerator or cupboard and prepare some food. They halfway chew it, swallow it, and expect it to be magically digested and assimilated. Our bodies are wonderful machines, but we often—albeit unknowingly—abuse them. We create stress on the digestive apparatus by eating anything and everything together. A favorite combination of foods for the "fast food connoisseur" is that of a hamburger, french fries and a Coke. Each of these foods is hard to digest to begin with, but the body has the additional burden of trying to separate each one for proper assimilation. The result is often constipation, stomachache and gas.

When we are young, we don't realize that these improper eating habits burden the body and gradually inhibit its ability to utilize the nutrients found in food. The gallbladder, liver, stomach, and large and small intestines suffer abuse until we finally feel the consequences of our decisions. Health-conscious people avoid junk food as much as possible, but some are unaware that there are certain combinations of natural foods which can also create havoc with digestion and vitality.

❖

This book explains the rationale behind proper food combining and ways to eliminate various digestion difficulties. It also examines how correct food combining, proper bowel management, and natural supplements can fortify the body against the ravages of chemicals, pesticides, herbicides, environmental pollution, etc. It also outlines natural approaches to ailments. This new knowledge will reinforce in you, the reader, the need for self-discipline and menu planning. You can change your life by choosing a healthier lifestyle! The *Nutritional Guide* is dedicated to all those who want to learn for themselves and are willing to apply the principles essential for ideal health.

Louise Tenney, M.H.

1

AUTOINTOXICATION

Let food be thy medicine.
Hippocrates

Hippocrates claimed that chronic disease comes from autointoxication, or self-poisoning due to constipation. Deposits of accumulated waste in the colon release toxins which inflame the nerves, producing rheumatism, neuralgia, melancholia, hysteria, eczema, acne, headaches, and many other health problems. Some contemporary natural health experts also believe that all sickness begins in the colon. Before World War II, doctors understood this concept and treated illness by giving enemas and colonics. This was before drugs and surgery gained a foothold as the supposed universal antidotes to disease.

Autointoxication creates an internal environment where germs and viruses can feed, multiply and flourish. Toxins can be passed on from mother to child before birth, and they can also accumulate from infancy throughout life. Toxemia and enervation (lowered resistance) greatly contribute to all types of chronic diseases. And chronic disease is "the beginning of the end" of slow poisoning caused by toxins in the body.

Faulty digestion also plays a role in autointoxication. If food is not digested properly, amino acids can be converted by microbes into powerful toxic substances such as phenol, indol, histidine, and indican. These toxins can cause symptoms such as fatigue, nervousness, gastrointestinal upsets, skin problems, headaches, insomnia, glandular and circulatory system disturbances, etc.

❖

Autointoxication also affects the functioning of both the liver and the brain. It poisons them via the bloodstream and can cause many problems; among them poor memory, personality changes and lower immunity. Autointoxication has also been linked to arthritis, breast disease, emotional disorders, and mental illness.

At the turn of the 20th century, Dr. J. A. Stucky, M.D., made this observation, "That blood is poisoned through absorption of toxic material from the intestinal canal more frequently than from any other source, I think will not be questioned." Toxins are manufactured daily in the intestinal canal and can also result from disturbed body chemistry. Irritated nerves and poisoned cells protest in the form of rheumatic pains, asthmatic attacks, vertigo, neuralgia, headaches and obscure neuroses of eye, ear, nose and throat. Medical literature has published reports over the years which support the theory of toxemia and disease.

❑ One doctor studied over 450 cases of allergies and found that they cleared up when intestinal toxemia was eradicated.

❑ Another doctor, after observing patients with asthma for 23 years, stated that toxemia is the root cause of the condition and that "the results of treatment justify my position."

❑ It has been discovered that approximately half of all cases of inflammatory arthritis can be greatly improved by removing the toxins formed in the intestine.

❑ About one-fourth of all cases of "irregular heartbeats" responded well to the elimination of toxemia.

❑ Several hundred cases of ear, nose and throat diseases reported in scientific literature were from autointoxication.

❑ Toxemia during pregnancy often stems from constipation and a high-protein diet.

❑ Many cases of eye disease and problems were improved when intestinal toxins were removed from the body.

❑ At a meeting of the American Medical Association in 1917, a report stated that 517 cases of mental problems were relieved by eradicating intestinal toxemia. These symptoms ranged from mental sluggishness to hallucinations. More recently, schizophrenia has been added to the list of mental disorders which improve when toxemia is eliminated.

❖

Norman W. Walker, D.Sc., Ph.D., has lectured and written extensively about toxemia. In his book *Colon Health,* he says: "If a person has eaten processed, fried and overcooked foods, devitalized starches, sugar and excessive amounts of salt, his colon cannot possibly be efficient—even if he should have a bowel movement two to three times a day! Instead of furnishing nourishment to the nerves, muscles, cells and tissues of the walls of the colon, such foods can actually cause starvation of the colon."

There is an opening in the cecum (part of the ascending colon) which plays a vital role in colon health. It is called the "ileocecal valve." The physiology text *Guyton* says: "A principal function of the ileocecal valve is to prevent backflow of fecal contents from the colon into the small intestine. Usually the valve can resist reverse pressure of as much as 50 to 60 centimeters of water." According to health author Dr. William F. Welles, this means "the valve is designed to resist considerable pressure before it lets fecal contents re-enter the small intestine . . . It is clear from this that the ileocecal valve is incompetent in the majority of Americans. As the ileocecal valve becomes incompetent, the contents of the large bowel back up into the no longer sterile environment of the small intestine, toxins enter the bloodstream, the liver becomes overburdened, and not only high cholesterol, but also autointoxication result."

PROPER ELIMINATION

The five organs of elimination are: the bowel, the kidneys, the lungs, the liver and the skin. The skin? Yes! It is often referred to as "the third kidney." In hot weather we drink more water and perspire through the skin more profusely. During cold weather we seem to drink fewer liquids and perspire less. Then we eliminate mainly through urination. When the skin is clogged by dead cells, soap accumulations and other matter, it cannot "breathe" properly. It is prevented from discharging toxins out of the body. This important eliminative channel can suffocate and trap waste materials, which otherwise would cleanse out through the pores. It is suggested by health experts that a daily "dry skin massage" is beneficial for this problem. Dr. Bernard Jensen, in his book *Beyond Basic Health,* says:

Brush for above five minutes before showering or taking a bath in the morning. Brushing the skin removes the uric acid crystals, catarrh, and other acid wastes that come up through the pores of the skin. I recommend this as "dry bathing." You can do it twice a day, if you desire.

We build new skin every day, and brushing the skin twice daily helps the body to eliminate, get rid of old skin cells, and keep pores open. Some patients told me they had begun to perspire again after skin brushing, when they hadn't been perspiring for years.

The keys to proper elimination through the five organs are daily exercise, proper diet (including herbs and supplements), positive mental attitude and stress control. Constipation results when the bowels are sluggish and the peristaltic movements do not function well.

CONDUCTING A CLEANSE

The human body was designed to operate at a very high level of health. However, due to the interference of various elements—faulty eating habits, emotional and physical stresses, environmental pollutants, daily intake of refined foods—this is not always possible. The body will, however, try to compensate for the imbalance created by these factors. It will adjust and adapt as much as possible until all avenues are exhausted and it succumbs to weakness and disease.

To restore health, a person must first cleanse, then build. The body will not readily accept the health-building properties of juices, fresh fruits and vegetables, or herbs if it is filled with toxins and mucus. Therefore, it is important to first clean the body of these barriers. We then strengthen the body with vitamins, minerals, herbs, enzymes, amino acids, etc., found in natural foods. The results are increased vitality, energy and zest for life. However, you do not have to wait until disease strikes to go on a cleanse. Everyone accumulates toxins through the years, and it is good to embark upon a periodic and thorough "housecleaning."

It is recommended that a person go on a juice fast anywhere from twenty-four hours to four days. To facilitate cleansing, an herbal enema is suggested. The following herbs cleanse the body: red clover, chaparral, echinacea, pau d'arco (taheebo), cascara sagrada, black walnut, goldenseal, burdock, devil's claw, fenugreek, gentian, Oregon grape and psyllium.

During a fasting period, fresh juices and homemade soups can be taken. They contain an abundance of nutrients that will assist in the detoxification of the body. Avoid using fluoridated water and aluminum pans and cooking utensils at all costs. During the first part of a fast you may notice that you experience flu-like symptoms or maybe even skin rashes or blemishes. Don't worry—this is nature's way of telling you that toxins are being released. It is a good sign and it will pass.

Dr. Norman W. Walker, an authority on juice fasting, explains that the safest way to fast is to take fruit juices for only three to four days at a time, and then to drink vegetable juices and eat raw vegetables and fruits for two to three days afterward. Juices that are freshly juiced have the most value during a cleasning fast. The following list discusses the advantages of various juices:

Beet Juice: Beets are blood builders. Their nutrients also nourish the lymphatic system, kidneys and bladder. Beets contain vitamins A, C, B complex, iron, calcium, potassium, phosphorus and sodium.

Carrot Juice: Carrots are very helpful for cleansing and nourishing. Less than a full cup of this fresh juice contains more than 30,000 units of vitamin A and an abundance of calcium. The juice assists in restoring balance within the intestinal tract.

Cabbage Juice: Cabbage is healing to the stomach tissues and helps encourage the appetite. Cabbage provides sulphur, calcium, iodine and vitamin U, which helps alleviate ulcers.

Cucumber Juice: Cucumbers contain silicon, calcium, potassium, sulphur, and vitamins B, B$_1$, B$_2$. It also helps equalize blood pressure.

Celery Juice: Celery juice helps clear the body of mucus. Celery's high calcium content feeds the nerves and alleviates insomnia. It is rich in natural sodium. This assists digestion and mobility of joints and tendons.

Apple Juice: The malic acid and glucose in apple juice are excellent for the nerves. Apple juice purifies the blood, helps regenerate health, and purifies the skin and other tissues. It provides vitamins A, B-complex and C. It also contains high amounts of potassium.

❖

PROGRAM

Modify this program to fit your needs. A weak person should only fast for one day, stronger individuals may fast from three days to a week. If a person is really weak, he or she should not fast at all because the body's energy is so depleted.

1. Upon rising, drink one glass of warm, pure water with the added juice of half a lemon. Throughout the day use other juices or pure water, as you become thirsty.

2. Twice a week in the afternoon or evening, use an herbal enema.

3. Take a brisk walk once a day for half an hour.

4. Try to forget your worries and stress.

2

PROPER DIGESTION

What happens to our food after it enters the mouth? There is a specific coordination of activities within the four parts of the body involved with digestion: the mouth and esophagus, the stomach, the small intestine and the large intestine.

The Mouth and Esophagus

You smell the wonderful aroma and your mouth starts watering. You taste the food and your saliva really starts to flow. You chew the food slowly and carefully because good chewing is vital for strong immune and digestive systems and for a healthy colon. Any disease can be improved when chewing is practiced in earnest. The healing process is accelerated when proper chewing is used in practice.

Why is chewing important? Solid foods cannot be broken down adequately in the stomach without proper chewing. Foods must be mixed with saliva. Saliva contains the digestive enzyme ptyalin, which changes complex carbohydrates into simple sugar, which in turn, converts to glucose. If we do not chew well, the ptyalin enzyme cannot permeate the grains and starch does not change into glucose. The stomach has no digestive juices to simplify carbohydrates so fermentation takes place if foods are not prepared by chewing. The result is excessive gas and discomfort in the stomach. Medications such as antihistamines and diuret-

✦

ics tend to dry the mucous membranes, which interferes with the secretion of the enzyme amylase (pepsin) and can alter the initial function of digestion. If this occurs, when food enters the stomach, digestion is already incomplete. This creates chronic gas and bloating, just as when food is not chewed well.

Saliva increases with chewing. There are three main pairs of salivary glands: 1) The parotid glands, located under the ears on both sides of the head, are much larger than the other glands and produce the greatest amount of saliva. Chewing helps to stimulate the parotid glands to produce a ptyalin-rich saliva. Salty and bitter foods also stimulate these glands. 2) The submaxillary glands are located along the side of the lower jawbone. They produce additional saliva needed for sour and oily foods, and for chewing meat. 3) The sublingual glands, found at the floor of the mouth, are smaller than the other glands. When we eat sweet foods or bite into fruits and vegetables, these glands produce a thinner saliva to dilute strong sweet tastes.

Each bite of food should be chewed 32 times. Chewing food properly helps our taste return to natural foods. Eating too fast destroys our ability to taste properly and enjoy natural foods. Chewing slowly also protects us from poisons, or toxic materials, by warning us of strange tastes. Chewing also helps us control our appetite. When we chew well, the stomach feels full when it is at only 80 or 90 percent of its capacity. To lose weight, chew your food three times as much.

When we swallow big pieces of food, use strong spices, eat too much sugar or salt, drink alcohol, coffee, very hot soup or tea, or eat in the middle of the night, we are indulging in improper eating habits. When we eat without chewing well, large pieces of food remain in the stomach for a long time and the stomach excretes more acid and creates fermentation—with its accompanying gas, burps, and belches. Then real stomach problems can begin.

Correct and thorough chewing also helps strengthen the teeth and gums. Saliva excretes a special hormone for maintaining strong teeth. This hormone, parotin, is only produced by the parotid glands through chewing. It is absorbed by the lymph vessels through the mouth during chewing, and then goes into the bloodstream where it stimulates cell metabolism and thus renews the entire body.

❖

The greatest benefit that chewing provides is increasing T-cell function. One of the special jobs of the hormone parotin is to stimulate the thymus gland, thereby producing more T-cells—a vital function in the immune system.

THE STOMACH

The stomach weighs approximately 4.5 ounces and an adult male can put five to eight pints into it (except for holidays and special occasions). It consists of "folds" that expand as food is introduced. Some people try to stuff as much as they can into their stomach out of habit, but it is best to stop eating before you are completely full. It takes more energy to digest food than any other bodily function. Therefore, the more food there is to take care of, the less energetic you will feel. Proteins and fats take longer to digest than grains, fruits or vegetables. If you don't want to fall asleep, eat lightly!

When food enters the stomach, four major digestive aids are produced: mucus, hydrochloric acid (HCL), pepsin (a protein-digesting enzyme), and gastrin (a hormone). In the stomach hydrochloric acid is responsible for breaking down the food, destroying germs and utilizing the pepsin. Too much hydrochloric acid causes stomach ulcers and too little increases the chances of developing gastric cancer. Excess hydrochloric acid is produced by anger, worry and anxiety and causes the stomach walls to become swollen and inflamed. A lack of HCL secretion in the stomach will influence the digestion of carbohydrates, fats, and protein.

Emotional stress plays a major role in stomach digestive disorders. The stomach is a very sensitive organ and nervous problems can slow down or speed up digestion. Under acute stress the stomach has a tendency to shut off acid production. Chronic stress causes an excessive excretion of hydrochloric acid, which can cause acid indigestion. This irritation of the mucous membrane lining of the stomach is what causes ulcers and hiatal hernia (a regurgitation reflex in the esophagus). It is a big mistake to eat while in this state of emotional stress. Only natural food should be eaten to create proper digestion.

SMALL INTESTINE

After the stomach does its churning, food moves into the duodenal areas of the small intestine. This is where food comes in contact with enzymes from the pancreas and bile system. The pancreas secretes enzymes for the digestion of carbohydrates, fats and protein, and it breaks down the nucleic acids RNA and DNA.

A buffer bicarbonate secretion created in this area of the colon will, if sufficient, neutralize the hydrochloric acid as it enters the small intestine from the stomach. Duodenal ulcers are created if there is not enough bicarbonate to act as a neutralizer.

The small intestine is the most important organ in proper digestion. It is where most of our nutrients are absorbed. It is also where water, salt, mucus and numerous enzymes are combined for absorption. The small intestine is so important that its loss would demand intravenous feeding. As long as we keep our small intestine in proper order, we continue to acquire nourishment to sustain life.

LIVER AND GALLBLADDER

The next important organs to help with digestion are the liver and the gallbladder, which secrete and store a substance called bile. Bile works to make solubles out of fats and helps neutralize hydrochloric acid. It also helps in the digestion of the fat-soluble vitamins A, D, E, and K. Bile salts stimulate the removal of waste products and various trace minerals in the body. Bile also promotes the normal peristaltic action of the colon so constipation can occur if the gallbladder is not functioning properly.

The concentrated bile from the gallbladder is stored between meals, but when meals are eaten the stored bile is released by contractions of that organ. If you don't have your gallbladder anymore, you can develop bloating and become deficient in vitamins A, D, E, and K. You may also have a constant dripping of bile from the liver all day long, so when meal times arrive there is not enough to digest the food properly. The constant drip irritates the small intestine which can cause colitis. If your gallbladder has been removed, it would be beneficial to drink a lot of water throughout the day as this will help dilute the constant drip of bile.

LARGE INTESTINE

When the digestive process is not functioning properly, the large intestine can be in trouble. If there has been faulty peristaltic action causing constipation, diverticulosis can result, putting fermented material in the pockets of the colon. Many health problems can originate as a result.

The rectum is the last link in the digestive system. This is where irritations, itching and hemorrhoids can develop. When a person becomes ill, the transit time of food is slowed. An enema or herbal laxative should be used to clean out the system.

DIGESTION DISTURBANCES

Bloating: Bloating can be due to liver and gallbladder sluggishness. Add lecithin, inositol, choline, and methionine (an amino acid), and B6.

Poor Digestion: Dr. W. A. Hemmings, an English allergist, feels that poor digestion of food can lead to the absorption of partially-digested food, which may in turn induce allergic reactions.

Flatulence: Flatulence increases when starting on a health diet and introducing too much new food at first, such as nuts, beans, cereals and other new foods. This is caused by gas-producing bacteria in the colon that metabolize the fiber content of the new foods. As your body becomes used to the new foods it will produce its own enzymes to help with gas problems. Always introduce new foods one at a time and in small amounts.

Weight Problems: A poor digestive system can cause obesity. When we do not completely digest certain fats and proteins they can be stored as body fat. When the body does not obtain what it needs, it constantly tries to obtain nutrients by creating a never-ending appetite. A vicious cycle ensues until the body is satisfied with enough nutrients.

MALABSORPTION

When the body is unable to absorb and metabolize nutrients from foods it is called "malabsorption." People whose bodies are not balanced and who do not digest their food properly may not be obtaining adequate nutrition. They may experience fatigue, irritability, moodiness and may complain of being unable to gain or lose weight. Both obese and underweight individuals need to evaluate their digestion to see if that is the problem. Stress, glandular imbalance and parasites may also play a role in these disorders. Proper food combining allows the digestive system to concentrate on one or two foods at a time and promotes balance in that system. Eating on a regular schedule and avoiding in-between-meal snacking are other ways to assist better digestive function.

The type of food a person eats can also alter their psychological outlook on life. Milk and sugar products provoke negative reactions in many people. Milk has been known to cause depression, feelings of helplessness and the inability to cope with everyday problems. Sugar can aggravate emotions such as despair, depression and alienation from others. Many times these symptoms can be linked to allergic reactions to these foods. Even wheat has caused emotional disorders. It is theorized that the use of pesticides and chemical fertilizers on wheat today could be part of the reason.

Overgrowth of the yeast organism *Candida albicans* is a common plague today. It can play a part in immune dysfunction, allergies, and even mental instability. A woman named Karen relates a problem she had with candida. She experienced psychological and emotional low times, and at one time even considered suicide. She yelled at her kids, didn't want her husband to come around her, and she caught every disease that came along. Her children were all born with thrush (which is caused by candida). Karen didn't know what to do. She seemed to always be sick, both emotionally and physically. Then one day she read an article on natural health. She went to the health food store and bought books on nutrition. She changed her diet by eliminating refined foods and exchanging them for whole foods. She still experienced indigestion and gas, however, until she began taking digestive herbs and eliminating meat from her diet. Karen finally found relief by taking acidophilus, which helped with the yeast. She also took vitamins, minerals, grains, raw seeds and nuts, and raw fruits and vegetables. Karen was able to change the negativities, both mental and physical, by changing her diet. She states, "I feel very positive about life now! My husband and I are closer now, and my relationship with my children is stronger. I feel more at peace than I ever have before."

FERMENTATION

Did you know that education is necessary for proper digestion? It is imperative that a person learn which foods are "digestion compatible." Different foods require different time schedules. Mixing "incompatible foods" will result in some of them digesting while others lie and rot in the digestive tract, because they require a longer digestive period and different enzymes. The result is gas, stomachache, and many times, a feeling of lethargy. In his book *Earning Good Health and Long Life,* health author Glen R. Shaw states, "Low energy and the need for extra sleep are sure signs that you need to change the food combinations you are eating." Mr. Shaw recounts an experience he had. "I can remember not long after I married, eating a lot of tuna fish sandwiches, and I soon went to the doctor complaining of gas. He gave me some charcoal pills and said I was swallowing too much air as I ate. The trouble, of course, was eating meat and bread together, along with salad dressing. The bread stopped digesting when the stomach changed the pH to digest the tuna fish. The improperly digesting bread then started forming gas."

Digestion is the first step to converting food to energy. The digestive tract provides our bodies with the essential nutrients for survival. Digestion does not all take place in the stomach. The mouth, stomach, and small intestine all help digest food. Also, in the colon there will be some residue of nourishment to be absorbed. If we had the ability to see inside our stomachs, we might be more careful what we carelessly dump into it. Good health depends upon our body's ability to properly digest and assimilate food, distribute nutrients from the food, and adequately eliminate waste from the bowels. Health author Lee DuBelle explains that:

• Acid fruit inhibits the flow of protein digestives.
• Different proteins, eaten at the same time, confuse the timing of when to send the strongest and weakest digestive juices.
• Fat inhibits the flow of protein digestives.
• Sweet fruits inhibit the flow of protein digestives.

THE CANDIDA CONNECTION

When fermentation occurs, sugars turn the undigested foods into an alcohol type composition. This promotes the unchecked growth of the yeast organism *Candida albicans.* The excessive alcohol content which results from fermentation and candida can actually make a person drunk! This sounds far-fetched, but it is true. Dr. John H. Jeffries, M.D., states:

> Production of large amounts of alcohol causes one to become a living "still." Production of large amounts of alcohol within the body causes even the nondrinker to become drunk . . . an overgrowth of *Candida albicans* in the gastrointestinal tract produces systemic biochemical changes and, for want of a better term, "phony's" the immune system. It also sends out "phony" signals to the glands, which cause the endocrine system to act as a free agent, without checks and balances. Alcohol is produced mainly by the fermentation of sugars and starches. (*Total Health,* June 1986)

Other contributors to the fermentation process are: 1) drinking fluids with meals, which dilutes hydrochloric acid (HCL) so that it cannot adequately breakdown food; 2) eating just before you go to bed, because digestion slows down or stops altogether at night; and 3) worry or negative emotions that affect proper digestion. Do not eat while you are upset because any food will turn to poisons in your system.

DIGESTION DESTROYERS

Aging: Our stomach produces less HCL as we grow older. We have also destroyed the enzymes that produce HCL by the foods we eat.

Alcohol: Produces acid, causing both a burning effect on the stomach lining and inflammation. This is why alcoholics have gastritis problems.

Antacids: Reduce HCL in the stomach and prevent protein from being digested. They will neutralize acids that are causing fermentation, but they also reduce the natural HCL production. More natural HCL is needed to treat the cause rather than the symptoms.

Antibiotics: Destroy the friendly bacterial flora in the colon. This causes deficiencies of the B-complex vitamins and vitamin K, and can lead to dysentery.

Chlorinated Water: Interferes with digestion. If digestion is a problem, change to pure water and the digestive formulas will work better.

Coffee: Increases acid production, especially black without cream as a buffer.

Cola Drinks: Contain phosphoric acid which signals the stomach that acid is already present, and it does not have to produce its own hydrochloric acid.

Diarrhea: Interferes with proper digestion and causes nutritional problems.

Liquids: Drinking liquids with meals dilutes HCL in the stomach so there isn't enough to digest food adequately.

Mineral Oil: Keeps B-complex vitamins from being absorbed in the body and destroys vitamin A.

Nitrosamines: Form in the stomach from two food constituents, amines and nitrites. Cancer of the bladder, esophagus and stomach increase when they are present. Nitrites are more likely to be formed with the lack of hydrochloric acid.

Processed Food: It is thought that one cause of gastric ulcers is processed food which lacks natural fiber and protein but is high in calories. Natural food is one of your best protections against stomach problems.

Stress or Worry: Reduce enzyme production so don't eat when you are worried or under stress. If you need to eat, eat only food that is easy to digest.

Improper Food Combining: Wrong combinations of food can create indigestion and acid stomach. Proper food combining means eating foods that will digest well together. Protein and starch are a poor combination. Sugars should not be consumed with proteins or starch and fruits should be eaten alone.

MORE FOOD FOR THOUGHT

Dr. William Donald Kelley, who was given the Humanitarian Award in 1975 by the International Association of Cancer Victims and Friends, says,

> No one in this society should eat protein without taking pancreatic enzymes at the same time. Pancreatic enzymes are the safest and cheapest insurance available against cancer. We find hydrochloric acid deficiencies very widespread, even among teenagers, so most people need this supplement, not just cancer patients. Moreover, among vegetarians hydrochloric acid deficiency is virtually universal. I've only found one vegetarian in all my years of practice who did not need this supplement.

Without proper digestion of food, assimilation and elimination of nutrients can seriously interfere with the proper function of the whole body. Minerals cannot be assimilated without sufficient hydrochloric acid in our stomach. Dr. Kelley says, "To make sure your body absorbs the minerals properly, take hydrochloric acid tablets. Since mineral absorption is so important for a healthy pancreas, you could also consider hydrochloric acid tablets to be a cheap form of anti-cancer insurance just like pancreatic enzyme tablets."

Food and stress are the root of digestive problems. The following list of ingredients are necessary in a good formula to increase the levels of HCL and to improve the assimilation of both vegetable and animal protein. There is probably no other combination of natural ingredients that can benefit the body more. The gastrointestinal system needs support and these are nutrients that help the body utilize the food for a healthy body and mind. A large part of our population cannot produce the proper amount of pancreatic digestive enzymes and adding this important supplement to the diet improves digestion and health.

Hydrochloric Acid: HCL is necessary for the assimilation of vitamins and minerals, especially vitamin C and calcium. It keeps bacteria under control. If the bacteria is not destroyed in the stomach, it will interfere with the absorption of food nutrients. One of the primary causes of an overacid stomach is the lack of HCL. When missing or in low supply it allows the food to ferment, thus causing acids of fermentation which are many times more damaging to the stomach. This fermentation of acids can cause ulcers and gallbladder attacks.

HCL has been proven very effective in killing harmful bacteria. When traveling and eating different and strange food and water, it should be a part of the daily diet. It has the ability to break down toxic elements. Professor A.E. Austin claims HCL to have strong germicidal properties. He says:

When hydrochloric acid content of the gastric fluid is deficient or absent, grave results must gradually and inevitably appear in human metabolism. First of all, we shall have an increasing and gradual starvation of the mineral elements in the food supply. The food will be incompletely digested and failure of assimilation must occur.

Secondly, a septic (pus forming toxins in the blood or tissues) process of the tissues will appear: pyorrhea, dyspepsia, nephritis, appendicitis, boils,

✧

abscesses, pneumonia, etc., will become increasingly manifested. Again, a normal gastric fluid demands activity of the gallbladder contents and of the pancreas for neutralization. Deficiency of normal acid leads to stagnation of these organs, causing diabetes and gallstones. In other words, an absence or a great deficiency of HCL gives rise to multitudinous degenerative reactions and prepares the way to all forms of degenerative disease.

Pepsin: Pepsin is a natural enzyme that breaks down proteins and is dependent on the HCL contents. It is secreted by the stomach when HCL is present. Pepsin breaks down protein into smaller components so it can be absorbed.

Pancreatin: This enzyme works as a catalyst for other protein digesting enzymes. It improves protein assimilation and helps digestion throughout the gastrointestinal tract.

Mycozyme: This enzyme also works as a catalyst and works with lipase and mylase in the digestion of fat and complex carbohydrates.

Papain: A powerful protein-digesting enzyme, papain is from the papaya fruit. Its purpose is to break down protein into amino acids. Papain contains proteolytic ferments which has the advantage of working in both acid and alkaline environments.

Bromelain: Bromelain is a natural vegetable enzyme from pineapple. It has the ability to digest protein for better absorption.

Bile Salts: These salts are essential for fat digestion. They stimulate the bile flow to combat constipation and improve gallbladder function. They are essential for fat absorption, including absorption of essential fatty acids and fat-soluble vitamins.

Lipase: Lipase is a natural aid in digestion of fat and complex carbohydrates.

3

NUTRIENTS FOR DIGESTION

To ensure proper digestion, certain nutrients are required by the body. This section will outline some of the most important nutrients, how they help in the process of digestion, and disorders that may result if there is a deficiency in the body.

Vitamin A: This vitamin promotes digestion and assimilation of food. Assists in maintaining normal glandular activity. Lack of vitamin A can cause digestive and intestinal disturbances and decreased gastric acid.

Acidophilus: This supplement increases friendly bacteria in the colon that are essential for the production of B vitamins. It helps to strengthen the immune system and reduces toxic wastes in the large intestines.

Aloe Vera: Stimulates peristalsis only on the lower third of the colon. This is very important to keep it clean and free from worms and parasites. It is very useful for the irritated colon, as found in colitis and Crohn's disease. It is helpful in cases of heartburn and other gastrointestinal disorders.

Lemon Juice: Lemon juice is metabolized in the body to an alkaline ash. Lemons assist in cleansing the stomach and liver. They are rich in potassium, vitamin C, bioflavonoids and calcium.

B-Complex Vitamins: Niacin stimulates the function of hydrochloric acid and the amino acid lysine. All the B-complex vitamins are involved one way or another in promoting a healthy digestive tract. They help with appetite stimulation, digestion, assimilation and elimination. They assist enzymes in metabolism of proteins, fats and carbohydrates. The B vitamins help sustain normal function of the gastrointestinal tract.

Vitamin C: Detoxifies nitrates and also destroys nitrosamines that have already been formed.

Calcium: A very important mineral. Decreased absorption of calcium is linked to low hydrochloric acid in the stomach, a deficiency that could lead to learning problems, hyperactivity and muscle spasms.

Catnip: This herb is "nature's Alka-Seltzer." Native Americans traditionally used it for infant colic. It is known to have a sedative effect on the nervous system.

Comfrey and Pepsin: This combination is very effective in dissolving the mucus coating in the small intestine, where absorption of nutrients takes place. A mucus coating is formed to protect the intestine from junk food, homogenized milk, pollutants and additives. The coating in the colon can become as tough and thick as plastic. Pepsin works on the mucus and comfrey helps hold the pepsin to the intestinal wall so it can dissolve the mucus. This formula is also a digestive aid. The allantoin content helps produce healthy new cells and is very nourishing.

Exercise: Very effective in helping the body produce lactic acid which improves digestion.

Fiber: Fiber foods assist the function and absorption ability of the intestinal tract. Whole natural foods, water and exercise are vital in maintaining the health of the digestive system.

Garlic: Neutralizes putrefactive toxins and kills bad bacteria. Eliminates gas and helps in digestion.

Gentian: Stimulates circulation and strengthens the system. It is usually used in digestive combinations for weakened muscular tone of the digestive organs.

Ginger: An excellent herb for indigestion as well as for stomach cramps. Ginger is very effective as a cleansing agent for the bowels and kidneys. It is good for circulation and promotes perspiration.

Goldenseal: Contains antiseptic properties and acts as a tonic on the mucous membrane lining of the stomach. Always use the herb in small amounts—it's more effective. Goldenseal is useful for digestive problems such as gastritis, peptic ulcers and colitis. If a person has low blood sugar it is wise to substitute myrrh instead of goldenseal.

Kefir and Yogurt: Both work to aid digestion. The lactic acid content acts as a cleanser and antiseptic for the gastrointestinal tract. All types of pathogenic bacteria and harmful germs are killed within five hours of eating these foods.

Magnesium: This mineral relaxes the gallbladder to help with pain and spasms. It aids in prevention of indigestion, alkalizes the system, reduces waste matter and helps elimination. Magnesium also calms nerves and activates enzymes.

Marshmallow: This relaxing herb will help reduce inflammation throughout the gastrointestinal tract.

Peppermint Oil: Excellent remedy for flatulence (gas). Add eight drops of oil of peppermint to one pint of water. A drop or two can be placed on the tongue for good results.

Psyllium Powder: Psyllium cleans the colon. When taken with a liquid it creates bulk and pulls toxins from the intestines and colon. It cleans the gastrointestinal tract to provide better digestion.

Water: Pure water helps keep the gallbladder stay healthy. Too little water can cause gallstones to develop, which are usually a combination of fats and calcium.

Zinc: Stimulates the digestive cells to release the compounds necessary for the conversion of digestive enzymes from the inactive form to the active form.

4

THE ROLE OF ENZYMES
AND AMINO ACIDS

ENZYMES

The word enzyme is derived from the word *enzymos* which means "ferment" or "leaven" (to make a change) in Greek. Enzymes are protein-like substances, formed in plants and animals, that are vital to health. They act as catalysts in chemical reactions to help speed up processes in the body which would normally take place very slowly or not at all. Glands and organs also depend upon enzymatic activity and cannot function properly without enzymes.

Enzymes exist in all living things. There are 700 different enzymes at work in the body and each one performs a different job. If the body is missing even one enzyme, there is a risk of failing health. But when we obtain enough enzymes from the food we eat, they help provide boundless energy. There are four main categories of food enzymes:

1. Lipase (serves to break down fat)
2. Protease (breaks down protein)
3. Cellulase (assists in breaking down cellulose)
4. Amylase (breaks down starch)

It is important to understand that enzymes can only be obtained from raw, live foods. A lack of such foods forces the body work hard to try and manufacture missing enzymes and overworks the glands. This can throw the glands out-of-balance and causes a person to feel fatigued and exhausted. This is why people who consume large quantities of cooked proteins and starches and very few enzyme-rich fruits and vegetables are often tired and have little energy. If we do not get sufficient enzymes, we will age faster. This is because our bodies' enzyme production slows down. Therefore, enzymes can be called the keys to the fountain of youth.

ENZYME KILLERS

☐ Fluoridated water paralyzes enzymes.
☐ Food cooked above 118 degrees kills live enzymes.
☐ Exposure to air and light dissipates enzymes. Pale, limp vegetables are enzyme-depleted foods.
☐ Long-term storage at room temperature or above diminishes enzymatic activity. Refrigerated food keeps a little longer, but it is best to eat food as fresh as possible. Sprouted beans, grains and seeds provide a treasure-trove of enzymes. Be sure to include plenty of fresh fruits, vegetables, their juices, and sprouted foods in your daily diet to ensure health and vitality!

AMINO ACIDS

Amino acids are the building blocks of proteins. A proper balance of amino acids can benefit the blood, the skin, the immune system and digestive system. Amino acids also can help with neurotransmitters in the brain, helping to stabilize moods and balance the thinking process. Health expert Carlson Wade observes, "A missing amino acid is like a missing building block. The entire structure may threaten to collapse because of a single weakness. For example, you may enjoy a corn-based diet, but corn is deficient in tryptophan, and this deficiency can cause emotional disorders and insomnia. If you add grains, seeds or nuts to corn, you will provide the tryptophan necessary for brain nourishment."

There are eight essential amino acids and twenty-four complementary ones which work synergistically to promote health throughout the entire body. Carnitine is an example of an amino acid which helps metabolize fat and reduce triglycerides. Carnitine is synthesized from the combination of the amino acids lysine and methionine. Methionine is an amino acid that helps remove heavy metals from body tissues.

THE PROTEIN MYTH

For many years—until recently, in fact—it was believed that you had to eat a complete protein at a meal in order for the body to utilize it properly. However, it has been discovered that if you eat complementary proteins throughout the day, the body will assimilate them and extract the amino acids it needs to regenerate its daily protein requirements for blood, enzyme, hormone and antibody production.

Most of the twenty-two amino acids needed for protein synthesis can be manufactured by the body. Eight cannot so they are called "essential" amino acids and must be supplied through diet. It is important to realize that the body can only utilize a measured portion of protein at any one time. Excess amino acids, whether from incomplete or complete proteins, are excreted in the urine. Therefore, a major portion of that big steak dinner is just a waste of money; it basically serves to gratify the taste buds.

There are many other myths which have been propagated throughout this century, primarily by those with vested interests in the food industry. Meat and dairy councils have financed advertising which heavily emphasizes animal products as major components of a healthy diet and good sources of protein. However, today commercial beef and chicken contain concentrated amounts of synthetic hormones, pesticides, antibiotics, etc., and these have harmful effects on the people who eat them. Proteins from plant sources, on the other hand, are more easily assimilated than the protein found in meats, which the body must arduously process in order to obtain any protein benefits. A person can experience more sustained energy from digesting fruits, vegetables, seeds and herbs than attempting to metabolize animal tissues.

Protein requirements for the body can be met if you obtain a sufficient amount of calories from a wide variety of vegetables, grains, legumes and fruits. Too much protein from animal-sources can leave toxic residues of metabolic wastes in the tissues as well as cause constipation, autotoxemia, hyperacidity, nutritional deficiencies, accumulations of uric acid, intestinal putrefaction, arthritis, gout, kidney damage, schizophrenia, atherosclerosis, heart disease and cancer. It can even contribute to premature aging and shorter life expectancy. Excessive protein in the diet can also cause a negative calcium balance which can pave the way for demineralization of bones or osteoporosis.

Complete proteins in a given day can be supplied by these combinations: corn and beans; rice and beans; grains and legumes; grains and seeds; or seeds and legumes. Of course, varying amounts of amino acids are found in most natural foods. Avoiding junk foods and concentrating on a nutritious diet will ensure that your body utilizes the protein efficiently.

Some people experience a craving for meat and interpret this feeling as their body's need for this type of food. People who stop eating red meat may experience withdrawal symptoms at first, but as their bodies release toxins, cravings will disappear. (Did you know that eating 12 ounces of char-broiled steak in one week is equivalent to smoking two packs of cigarettes a day for that same period?) If you cannot stop eating meat completely, try eating it sparingly as a complement to your meals rather than as the dominating food. The Asians are, as a group, very healthy. Maybe it is because their diets include plentiful amounts of grains and vegetables with little meat. Besides the fact that a high-meat diet is detrimental to health, it is also more expensive on the grocery bill. For delicious meatless recipes, refer to my book *Today's Healthy Eating*.

Acid/Alkaline Balance

According to health expert Dr. William Howard Hay, acid to alkaline foods should be balanced in a 1:4 ratio. Alkaline foods include all vegetables and fruits (except plums and cranberries), almonds, and sprouts from seeds, grains and beans. Acid foods include animal proteins such as meat, fish, shellfish, eggs, cheese and poultry. Other acid foods are nuts (except almonds) and foods made from cereal starches and sugars.

Though it is recommended that protein and starch foods are not included in the same meal, nature combines these two substances proportionately in grains, seeds and vegetables in a manner that is digestible. It is not good to eat proteins and starches in the same meal because they are in a concentrated form and do not assimilate well together. This is because proteins require an acid medium for digestion, and carbohydrates (starches and sugars) need an alkaline medium for this purpose. An improper combination upsets the digestive system and causes gas, bloating and a lethargic feeling.

CHOLESTEROL

The human body needs cholesterol. In fact, the body manufactures cholesterol from natural oils and fats that are ingested. The body is able to synthesize cholesterol for important purposes, but keeps the amountunder control by manufacturing lecithin. Lecithin is a "cholesterol regulator" that the body makes from nutrients in the diet. In nature, lecithin and cholesterol always accompany each other. An egg contains both of these substances, each keeping the other in balance.

Cholesterol serves many important functions: it helps build cell walls, assists in the synthesis of pituitary and sex hormones, and is used by the adrenal glands. The brain and the myelin sheaths that protect the nerves also require choledsterol. (Almost 25 percent of all the cholesterol in the human body is contained in the brain and spinal cord). Cholesterol is also made into bile acids to help metabolize fats and fat-soluble vitamins. Vitamin D can be synthesized in the body from cholesterol and assists in the metabolism of calcium.

THE CHOLESTEROL SCARE

The big "cholesterol scare" is the result of a distortion of information. There is no correlation between eating cholesterol-rich foods and blood cholesterol levels. These levels are entirely dependent upon the body's ability to take care of it through the liver; gallbladder and bowels. Sue Moody, author of *Cholesterol Confusion: Who is Responsible*, states:

> How did our ancestors and their ancestors survive and thrive on a diet filled with such foods as lard, eggs, butter and red meats? If the fat in the diet is the reason for high cholesterol and the cause of heart disease, then our civilization would not be in existence today, because before the third decade of this century the daily diet consisted almost entirely of animal fats, and cholesterol-rich foods. Heredity may be a major factor of high cholesterol and if this be the case, the amount of dietary cholesterol ingested

would have no correlation whatsoever on lowering the cholesterol levels in the blood.

Eight foods that have been shown to lower cholesterol are eggplant, garlic, fiber, apples, beans, yogurt, oat bran, and psyllium. Other foods and supplements which help are: salmon oil, evening primrose oil, olive oil, kelp, skullcap, goldenseal, hawthorn berries, barley, carrots, cayenne pepper; onions and lecithin.

Another health writer, David Skousen, explains, "Cholesterol is harmful if, instead of lubricating the walls of the body's blood vessels, it begins to stick to them and build up fatty deposits that also injure the sides of the vessel walls." To keep cholesterol in a safe condition, the body is able to create a substance that emulsifies cholesterol. In other words, it is broken up and dispersed so that it won't coagulate and adhere to artery walls. This naturally-occurring substance, called phospholipids, is a mixture of phosphorus and lipid fats. Another name is lecithin.

Excessive sugar intake can produce high triglyceride levels even in a healthy individual. Mr. Skousen explains it this way:

> The most abundant lipid of animal tissues is the triglyceride, but when people consume too many simple carbohydrates (sugar), they flood into the blood, requiring the liver to convert them into a triglyceride type of fat. These fats are called triglycerides because the liver hooks three fatty acids (tri) to a sugar or glycerine molecule (glyceride). However, too many of these thicken the blood and they can pile up and block capillaries or even arteries leading to vital tissues.
>
> There are two or three different forms of triglycerides, depending on who does the dividing. The body packages them with cholesterol and protein so they can ride the bloodstream better since water and oil don't mix.
>
> These packages are named lipoproteins. The biggest package has the very lowest density (VLDL). The middle package has a low density (LDL). But the smallest has the highest density of all (HDL), a very strange arrangement of opposites.
>
> VLDL packages carry most of the triglycerides in the blood and seem to be the most dangerous to artery health. LDL and HDL packages carry most of the cholesterol. It was finally discovered that those with the highest blood HDL's had the fewest heart attacks. Surprisingly, this had been

known by scientists for over 35 years, but hardly anybody gave it any attention! This was because cholesterol phobia branded its carrier as the bad boy. It was a case of guilt by association. Yet currently, HDL's are in.

Excessive cholesterol can be eliminated from the blood via bile that is discharged through the gallbladder into the bowels. It can either be reabsorbed into the blood, or the body will excrete it. The reabsorbed cholesterol can be metabolized by cells and reduced to carbon dioxide and water. Obviously, the body has its own method for balancing cholesterol levels as long as it is kept well-nourished, and the organs are functioning properly.

5

DIGESTIVE DISORDERS

ALLERGIES

Many people cannot enjoy eating certain foods because they are allergic to them. What causes sensitivities to foods? Some experts believe that when a specific type of food is the main component of a diet, that the body develops a peculiar reaction to it. The substances to which the body is sensitive are called allergens because they provoke the allergic response. It is believed that allergens irritate the system because they are made up of protein molecules which are bigger than those found normally in foods.

When blood vessels and mucous membranes are healthy, they screen out the larger protein molecules. They are able to do this because of their fine-knit structures. However, the blood vessel and membrane tissues of an allergic person are poor quality and allow the entry of the larger protein molecules. When the tissues of the body are irritated by these allergens, the body releases a chemical known as a histamine. This substance causes the mucous membranes to swell, and if the irritation is extensive, the entire body can be affected with subsequent swellings of the arms, legs, etc. Allergies have been linked to the usual red eyes and sniffles, but also to mental illness, fatigue, insomnia and a host of gastrointestinal disorders.

Allergic reactions are associated with lowered immune system function. Normally, the T-cells of the immune system take care of unwanted "invaders." When the immune system is not operating efficiently, the T-cells may be small in number or they are unable to recognize invaders from normal substances so they attack everything. When there is chaos in the immune system, allergies can be one of the results. Health expert Paavo Airola, Ph.D., has stated:

> The solution for digestive problems caused by allergies is as simple as it is difficult to implement: all allergens must be eliminated from the diet for a certain period, which must often extend for years, to give the body time to "forget" about them. Fasting is an excellent way to begin the treatment. Prolonged juice fasting, or repeated short fasts, will eventually result in better tolerance of previous allergens. After juice fasting, the patient can try a "mono diet," one food, which he knows he tolerates well, at a time. Then he can add one new food each week, testing it for a week. If the body's reaction is good, this food is kept in the diet and another new food is added—if the reaction is bad, that food should be discarded and a new food tried. This way all real allergens can be eliminated from the diet.

Stress can lower immunity and resistance to disease. It can also wreak havoc in the digestive system. There is a true story of an army surgeon from the 1700s, William Beaumont, who noticed a wound in a patient's stomach that did not heal after several weeks. The inquisitive surgeon used a glass rod to touch the inside of the man's stomach and observe the metabolic reactions to digestion and stress. Dr. Beaumont recorded that "the lining of the stomach had a soft, or velvet-like appearance With fear, anger, or whatever depresses the nervous system, the villous coat of the stomach becomes red and dry, at other times pale and moist."

Food addictions and binges are part of the food allergy syndrome. Author Annemarie Colbin explains in her book *Food and Healing:*

> We are addicted to a food or drink (and thus crave it) when A) the food creates symptoms of imbalances, such as headache, fatigue, skin problems, digestive disorders, or tension, some time after ingestion, and B) the symptoms can be relieved by consuming more of the same food. If, for example, you give up sweets or coffee, you will initially crave them and feel generally depressed and tense. Eat a cookie, have a cup of coffee, and the symptoms go away—although not the addiction.
>
> A food allergy is the opposite of addiction: Unpleasant symptoms appear almost immediately upon consumption of the offending substance and are

best controlled by avoiding that substance completely. There are many instances, however; when we do not connect our allergic symptoms with our food intake. We'll continue to crave the allergen and suffer through fatigue, tension and headaches without realizing what their cause is or how simply they could be cured.

Cravings for foods are caused by the body trying to correct imbalances. If we consume too many alkaline-forming foods, the body will manifest the imbalance by a craving for acid-forming foods. Cravings for the opposite, or complementary, foods do not always show up for foods with high nutritional value. Sometimes the cravings are for sugary sweets, coffee, alcohol or other detrimental foods. (You have probably read about kids who will eat dirt because their bodies are lacking some of the trace minerals which are found in soil.) The key to avoiding allergies is a varied diet with plenty of nutrients. The Chinese call the balance in the body "yin and yang." They are taught from childhood which foods are yin and which foods are yang, and when there is an imbalance in the body they instinctively eat the foods that have the balancing effect. The following list includes various gastrointestinal disorders associated with food allergies:

Celiac Disease: This disease has been connected to sensitivity to wheat gluten, soybeans, eggs and milk. Some experts feel that the gluten intolerance may be triggered by ingestion of cow's milk during infancy, which has permanently damaged the intestinal tract.

Crohn's Disease: This is a severe illness, characterized by colon inflammation. It has also been linked to gluten intolerance. Foods with even the tiniest bit of gluten must be eliminated from the diet.

Colitis: Allergens which are known to provoke colitis include milk, eggs, chocolate, meat, nuts, wheat, corn and citrus foods. There are cases of chronic ulcerative colitis which have gone into remission when dairy products were eliminated from the diet.

Colic: Infant colic has been eradicated when cow's milk has been eliminated from the breast-feeding mother's diet.

Hiatal Hernia: In his book *Hiatal Hernia Syndrome: Insidious Link to Major Illness,* Dr. Theodore A. Baroody explains:

Large portions of the population experience this disorder at one time or another in their lives—I estimate as high as 85 percent. It is an insidious masquerader that paves the way to many other serious disorders. I call it the Hiatal Hernia Syndrome. Hiatus is the special hole in the diaphragm, the breathing muscle, through which the esophagus normally passes to become the stomach. Hernia is the term for a weakened—in this case, stretched—muscle. If, for any reason, the diaphragmatic muscle is weakened or torn, the stomach will be forced upward through the diaphragm, creating the problematical condition.

Hiatal hernias cause all types of digestive disorders, including: regurgitation, vomiting, bloating, diarrhea, belching, hiccups, nausea, heartburn, and colic in children, plus many other symptoms.

6

THE HEALTHY WAY TO EAT

Fruit in the Morning

Fresh fruits are the cleansers of the body. Their high water content helps wash many toxins and impurities out of the system. The live enzymes in fruit also facilitate digestion and promote energy in the body. However, if combined with other foods they are unable to pass through the system as they were designed to do. They cause fermentation, indigestion and gas. Cooked fruit promotes an acid condition in the body, and thus becomes an acid-forming food. (Do not confuse acid foods with acid-forming foods.) Some acid foods (such as fresh fruit) actually help neutralize acidity in the body, as they become alkaline-forming once they are inside.

It takes more energy for the body to digest foods than to perform any other function. In the morning you need all the energy you can muster to start your day! Therefore, it makes sense that you eat a fruit meal, or drink fresh fruit juice for easy digestion and energy for morning demands. All fruit in season and all tree-ripened fruit contain the nutrients the human body needs to sustain itself.

Do not clog your body with hard-to-digest proteins and carbohydrates. During the period of time during the night when your body is without food it goes through a cleanse. This is when healing takes place because the body's energies can be directed to that instead of to digestion. Our bodies go through a type of fast while we sleep. When we eat in the morning we break our fast, hence, the name breakfast.

Toxins accumulate in the stomach and your first food in the morning should be a cleansing food. As mentioned in this book, take half of a fresh lemon squeezed in a glass of water; one hour or more before breakfast. Some people, such as those with hypoglycemia, diabetes or candida, cannot handle large amounts of fructose. Those with serious candida problems should avoid all fruit until further healing takes place. Some people who have had severe reactions to fruit find that it is the spray on the fruit, rather than the fruit itself, that cause the problem. People who cannot handle large quantities of fruit should start out slowly with fruit in the morning. It is suggested that they eat half of a fruit such as a banana or apple, and see how it is tolerated. Persons with the above conditions should avoid fruits with high sugar content, such as grapes and dried fruit (raisins and dates).

Nutritionists Harvey and Marilyn Diamond remind us in their book *Fit for Life* that "the human body is not designed to digest more than one concentrated food in the stomach at the same time. Any food that is not a fruit and is not a vegetable is concentrated."

Why do you get sleepy after a protein and carbohydrate meal? Try eating a fruit meal and then taking a nap. Do you see the difference? You can reach your own conclusion about which one helps you stay awake.

VEGETABLES AND PROTEIN FOR LUNCH

I do not advocate staying away from meat completely. However; meat should be a complementary, rather than a dominating, food in combination with vegetables. In other words, vegetables should constitute the major portion of the meal. They should be raw or lightly steamed. A vegetable salad with chicken or tuna is delicious! Or try your hand at Asian cooking. The Chinese have realized for years the benefits of this type of eating.

There are many variations to the vegetable/protein approach. You need not become bored. For mouth-watering sample dishes, turn to the recipe section in this book.

Vegetables and Grains for Dinner

Vegetables and grains are very compatible. Vegetables contain all of the body-building minerals needed for the body. It can synthesize some vitamins, but we must obtain minerals from our foods. Grains contain amino acids, minerals and supply roughage or fiber. This is very important for the health of the colon and entire digestive system.

Some people are sensitive to the gluten in wheat. Health expert Bernard Jensen, D.C., Ph.D., suggests that rice (which is gluten-free), rye (which builds muscle), and cornmeal (also gluten-free) are excellent grains. He says that "one of the finest wheat substitutes is millet. When I went to the Hunza Valley, I found these old men who died at 120 with every tooth in their head. They had plenty of calcium, and they were living on a lot of millet."

Food Combining

We have been taught that a balanced diet is one that includes many different foods at one meal, but actually that is an imbalanced meal. Too many different foods at one time can cause poor absorption, improper digestion, fermentation in the colon, heartburn, gas, and the formation of toxins. Simple preparation of food will assure proper digestion, assimilation and elimination.

Proper food combining starts with a glass of water with a half of lemon first thing in the morning. This cleans the stomach and helps the liver to get into action. Fresh fruit, cereal, seeds, or nuts can be eaten later on for breakfast. Lunch can consist of a fresh vegetable salad, nuts, vegetables, and rice. A fresh salad, steamed vegetables and baked potatoes are delicious for supper. It is best if no protein foods are eaten after 2 p.m. It is hard for the body to digest protein in the evening and it can cause fermentation. The following are guidelines for healthy eating and proper food combining:

❑ Eat acids and starches at separate meals.
❑ Eat protein foods and carbohydrate foods at separate meals.
❑ Eat but one concentrated protein food at a meal.
❑ Eat proteins and acids at separate meals.

❑ Eat fats and proteins at separate meals.
❑ Eat sugars and proteins at separate meals.
❑ Eat starches and sugars at separate meals.

Even though it is recommended that protein and starch foods are not blended in the same meal, nature skillfully combines these two substances proportionately in grains, seeds, and vegetables in a manner which is digestible. When man eats proteins and starches in the same meal, they are in a concentrated form and do not assimilate well together. This is because proteins require an acid medium for digestion, and carbohydrates (starches and sugars) need an alkaline medium for this purpose. An improper combination upsets the digestive system and causes gas and bloating and a lethargic feeling.

High-protein foods and grains are usually acid-forming foods. There must be a balance between acid-forming foods and alkaline-forming foods in the diet. According to health expert Dr. William Howard Hay, acid to alkaline foods should be balanced in a 1:4 ratio. Alkaline foods include all vegetables and fruits (except plums and cranberries) and almonds. Acid foods include animal proteins (meat, fish, shellfish, eggs, cheese, poultry, nuts (except almonds); also food made from cereal starches and sugars). Most nutritionists agree that it is wise to eat milk products by themselves.

The above may scare you into thinking, "What can I eat?" However, the following are easy charts to which you can refer.

Easy Food Combining

Certain types of foods can be eaten together. There are, however, some food combinations that are best avoided.

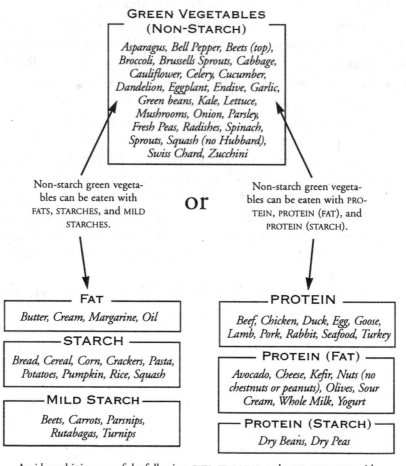

Green Vegetables (Non-Starch)

Asparagus, Bell Pepper, Beets (top), Broccoli, Brussells Sprouts, Cabbage, Cauliflower, Celery, Cucumber, Dandelion, Eggplant, Endive, Garlic, Green beans, Kale, Lettuce, Mushrooms, Onion, Parsley, Fresh Peas, Radishes, Spinach, Sprouts, Squash (no Hubbard), Swiss Chard, Zucchini

Non-starch green vegetables can be eaten with FATS, STARCHES, and MILD STARCHES.

or

Non-starch green vegetables can be eaten with PROTEIN, PROTEIN (FAT), and PROTEIN (STARCH).

Fat
Butter, Cream, Margarine, Oil

Starch
Bread, Cereal, Corn, Crackers, Pasta, Potatoes, Pumpkin, Rice, Squash

Mild Starch
Beets, Carrots, Parsnips, Rutabagas, Turnips

Protein
Beef, Chicken, Duck, Egg, Goose, Lamb, Pork, Rabbit, Seafood, Turkey

Protein (Fat)
Avocado, Cheese, Kefir, Nuts (no chestnuts or peanuts), Olives, Sour Cream, Whole Milk, Yogurt

Protein (Starch)
Dry Beans, Dry Peas

Avoid combining any of the following: FATS, STARCHES, and MILD STARCHES, with any of the following: PROTEIN, PROTEIN (FAT), and PROTEIN (STARCH). Fermentation will occur.

┌─ SWEET, DRIED FRUIT ─┐

Apricot, Banana, Date, Fig, Peach, Pear, Pineapple, Prune, Raisins

┌─ SWEET, FRESH FRUIT ─┐

Banana, Black Currant, Mango, Papaya, Persimmon, Grape

┌─── SUGAR ───┐

Brown Sugar, Honey, Malt, Maple Syrup, Molasses, White Sugar

┌─── MELON ───┐

Cantaloupe, Casaba, Crenshaw, Honeydew, Muskmelon, Watermelon

Fruits in each of these categories need to be eaten alone because they require different digestive enzymes in order to be assimilated. Do not eat fruit with any other types of foods. Milk is to be ingested separately from all foods. Sugars are to be eaten alone.

┌─── FRUIT (ACID) ───┐

Acerola Cherry, Apple (sour), Cranberry, Currants, Gooseberries, Grapefruit, Sour Grapes, Kumquats, Lemons, Limes, Loganberries, Oranges, Pineapple, Plum (sour), Pomegranate, Tangerine, Tomato

┌─ FRUIT (SUB-ACID) ─┐

Apple, Apricot, Blackberries, Blueberries, Boysenberries, Cherries (sweet), Nectarine, Peach (sweet), Pear, Plum, Raspberries

┌─── MILK ───┐

Eat separate from everything else

DIGESTION TIME

The digestion time of various foods is determined by how easy they are to assimilate by the body. Foods which are easily digested are often referred to as "mild foods" since they do not require a lot of work and energy to digest. The following are approximate time tables for digestion:

Green vegetables (non-starch)	5 hours
Raw juices	15 minutes
Fat	12 hours
Protein (meat)	12 hours
Protein (fat)	12 hours
Protein (starch)	12 hours
Starch	5 hours
Mild starch	5 hours
Fruit, sweet/dried	3 hours
Fruit (acid)	2 hours
Fruit (sub-acid)	2 hours
Fruit, sweet/fresh	3 hours
Melon	2 hours
Syrup, sugar	2 hours
Milk	12 hours

Weight Loss and Food Combining

Overloading the stomach and wrong food combining are the major causes of weight gain and obesity. Incorrect food combining is also the major cause of most diseases. In fact, many people are finding that their digestive troubles—their ailing gallbladders, malfunctioning livers, or disordered intestines—have been acquired because of improper food combining.

Nature cannot be fooled. If you eat large meals day in and day out and combine wrong foods, your stomach is bound to enlarge and stretch to two or three times its normal size. There are natural laws we must obey in order to have good health and normal weight. The body cannot handle wrong chemical conditions that disrupt normal digestion. If you eat too much of a certain kind of food, the digestive system has to overwork and the tissues connected with it can become inflamed. This sometimes takes a long time, over a period of years, but it will show wear and tear on the organs and tissues.

It is possible to build up a tolerance to incompatible mixtures of food. This is what most of us have done who have not been trained in proper eating habits. This leads to depletion of energy and does damage to the tissues and organs of the body. This weakens our whole system and causes us mental and physical diseases, which are very common.

Weight loss is the reward we achieve when we properly combine our food, and eat less. We have more energy, and as we gain this energy it gives us the desire to eat properly. This type of weight loss is gradual and permanent.

7

HERBS VS. DRUGS

Modern medicinal treatments are rapidly losing credibility. Drugs focus on a disease only after it invades the body and they create havoc with the immune system. There are too many adverse reactions to pharmaceutical drugs and antibiotics are now used so commonly that viruses and bacteria have built resistance to some some of them. The widespread use of vaccinations and antibiotics is considered one of the main causes of immune system disorders. Dr. Robert Mendelsohn has said, "There is a growing suspicion that immunization against relatively harmless childhood diseases may be responsible for the dramatic increase in autoimmune diseases since mass inoculations were introduced."

Autoimmune diseases are the epidemic plagues of our times. A large part of the population of the United States suffers from one or more of these disorders chronically. As long as we play games with the immune system and interfere with the body's only protection, we will see more and more unusual autoimmune diseases than we ever would have dreamed possible.

Another problem with current medical practices is that many of them simply do not work. A pamphlet put out by the government entitled *Assessing the Efficacy and Safety of Medical Technologies* says, "It has been estimated that only 10-20 percent of all procedures currently used in medical practice have been shown to be efficacious by controlled trial."

❖

(This pamphlet can be obtained from the U.S. Office of Technology Assessment for Publication #PB286-929.)

Organized medicine is virtually a monopoly. Its members are quick to silence, discredit and destroy people or organizations who offer approaches that do not ring up profits for its interests. The concern is that organized medicine ultimately seeks to outlaw our freedom of choice. They are trying to take our constitutional rights away from us. (For more information read *Proving Orthodox Medicine is Unproven,* put out by Coalition for Alternatives in Nutrition and Healthcare, Inc.)

Organized medicine attacks any alternate health care by accusing it of quackery. According to their own definition, if orthodox medicine is 80 percent unproven then they themselves are quacks! I believe the American Medical Association (AMA) should be more humble in their approach to what is either valid or quackery in the field of nutrition. It is a well-known fact that the medical doctors lack nutritional education. Why should the AMA be permitted to manipulate the government to prosecute alternative health care professionals who are helping people find better health and happiness? Most of us in the health field are not against medical doctors. In fact, we are grateful for them and have used them many times. We just want the freedom to choose the type of health care we choose.

I have heard the medical profession say if someone uses herbs they are self-diagnosing and the public is not capable of self-diagnosis. They say we are not capable of knowing what our bodies need. Some doctors have called herbs primitive and backwards, and drugs advanced and modern. Yet there are birth defects caused by using drugs. Is this advancement in medical technology? Have you ever heard of birth defects from using herbs?

Some doctors say that herbal treatments are really an uncontrolled form of drug therapy, that they are drugs because the average herb contains five or six drugs. Scientists have confirmed that whole herbs in their natural state are compatible to the body system and are accepted as food. We know that many drugs are derived from herbs. The problem arises when they remove part of an herb and do not use the part that prevents side-effects. The whole herb is designed to work together. I want to mention at this time that herbalists use only the herbs that are good

❖

for the body. Herbs are easily utilized to strengthen and balance, and nourish the body system and are completely eliminated, leaving behind health-building properties. The body has the knowledge to take from the herbs what it needs and disregard the rest, without side effects. The body does not know drugs, that is why there are so many side effects.

DRUGS AND THEIR SIDE EFFECTS

Many modern drugs powerfully and quickly help remove the symptoms of disease. This action usually only gives temporary relief but there are times when we need this quick action. At least we need to have a free choice in deciding what action we will take. The major problem is that drugs lead to more serious diseases later, as can also cause serious side effects. They are foreign substances to the human body. When a child is vaccinated, the body usually tries to eliminate the vaccine quickly by creating a fever; which is how the body eliminates foreign material. Drugs will not assimilate into the body's health-building metabolism. The body finds it hard to get rid of them once they are there. They accumulate in various organs and tissues to continue their negative side-effects.

HOW SAFE ARE DRUGS?

In January 1995, *U.S. News and World Report* carried an article on the danger of various drugs. It told about Marcy Behrendt 23 years of age, who in 1994 suffered a series of ministrokes that her neurologist suspects were caused by Norplant, the five-year contraceptive implanted in her arm the year before. Norplant was approved in December 1990, and in 1993 alone over 280,000 prescriptions were written, amounting to sales of 102 million dollars. Norplant's labeling now lists stroke among the possible side effects, and Marcy is currently taking stroke medication.

In another case, the drug Estrace was prescribed in 1992 for Sey Simpson, a schoolteacher, as part of estrogen replacement therapy. She was later hospitalized with severe pancreatitis. She is now disabled and has sued Mead Johnson, claiming a failure to warn of pancreas problems in people with high triglyceride levels. A revised label now includes that warning. Over four million prescriptions were written for this drug in 1993 for total sales of 65 million dollars.

❖

Another casualty of a dangerous drug was Christopher Tyson, 17 years old. He was given a Duragesic pain patch after dental surgery and he died that night in his heated water bed. The label did not warn that applying heat speeds the rate of drug release. Users are now told to avoid electric blankets and heating pads. In 1993, 500,000 Duragesic patches were prescribed for total sales of 83 million dollars.

Yet another lesson of the danger of drugs can be learned from Keith Slaten of Lonoke, Arkansas, age 34. Keith had to have a total hip replacement and a doctor told him that Prednisone, a drug he had taken intermittently his whole life for severe asthma, may have been responsible. In a lawsuit against two firms, he claims the label inadequately warns of the risks. The drug makers deny the charge. Prednisone is used for many disorders, including asthma and rheumatic disorders. Twelve million prescriptions worth 16 million dollars were written in 1993. The drug was approved in the mid 1950s (*Dangerous Drugs*, 48-53).

Medical care is a business that spends billions on treatments and drugs that have never actually been tested to determine their efficacy. We the mass population are their guinea pigs. We are the ones that do the testing and where the final results can cause crippling, pain, misery and even death. I will now discuss some of the other commonly used drugs that can have serious and sometimes dangerous side effects.

Prozac is a widely prescribed drug for depression. But how safe is it? Side effects from taking this anti-depressant range from: skin rash, itching, headache, nervousness, insomnia, drowsiness, tremors, dizziness and fatigue to impaired concentration, altered taste, nausea, vomiting, diarrhea, sexual impairment, fever, weakness, joint pain and swelling, swollen lymph glands, and fluid retention. Even more serious, this drug has recently been linked to suicide attempts and murders. It is believed to induce violent and persistent suicidal and homicidal tendencies in many people who otherwise would not even contemplate such behavior.

Another commonly used drug is Ritalin, a so-called quick solution to restlessness and hyperactivity in children. Ritalin has been dubbed "the behavior pill." Its slang names include qualudes, soupers and 714-ludes. Possible side effects may be stunted growth, seizures in children prone to them, blurring of vision, nervousness, insomnia, skin rashes and nausea. Even with the possible side effects, this drug is commonly prescribed.

❖

One woman said her son's teacher badgered her until she agreed to take her son to a doctor. The physician put the boy on Ritalin in the day and an antidepressant by night, but the behavior of this boy did not change. Additionally, his grades plummeted and he developed suicidal tendencies.

Remember when interferon was shouted as a miracle drug for cancer? It is a natural immune system chemical that the body produces itself. Interferon enhances the body's own defensive and healing mechanism, and is a stress and disease resistance factor. It was said to be especially effective as a protective factor against cancer, so drug companies began producing interferon artificially. But now we know that interferon is another chemical drug that backfired. Artificial interferon has proven very disappointing, showing anticancer action in only 10 to 20 percent of cancer patients, the results usually being temporary.

What we learn from this is that what is naturally produced by the body cannot be produced synthetically. A study released on April 19, 1982 showed that artificial interferon may increase the ability of cancer cells to spread into normal tissues. A natural alternative is vitamin C, which helps to produce natural interferon in the body. Many herbs contain large amounts of vitamin C. One recent study showed that licorice root actually stimulates the interferon production in the body. Kelp, burdock, capsicum, pau d'arco, red clover, chaparral and other herbs also help to protect the immune system.

Clomid is another chemical drug that the medical profession praises. It is used as a fertility medicine in some women who are unable to become pregnant. It is available only with a doctor's prescription. The directions say that it is very important that your doctor check your progress at regular visits, since you must stop taking this medicine if you become pregnant. A little scary, isn't it? This medicine may cause vision problems, dizziness or lightheadedness. It has caused personality changes in some women. It is now found that some women on Clomid (another human experiment) are thrown into premature menopause.

A drug called Bendectin, widely prescribed for pregnancy morning sickness, was pulled off the market because it was found to cause birth defects. The company that manufactured it was sued. A wide variety of fetal skeletal defects and other abnormalities were reported among the offspring of mothers using this drug.

Methapyrilene, an ingredient found in hundreds of nonprescription cold remedies and sleep-aid remedies, has been found to be a dangerous cancer-causing agent. The products that contain this substance include Nytol, Compoz, Sominex, Allerest and Excedrin P.M. This finding comes from the researchers at the Frederick Cancer Research Center in Maryland.

Another unsafe drug, dioxin, has been in the news many times. Scientists estimate that if efficiently administered, an ounce of dioxin could kill one million people. Dioxin is a by-product of chlorinated phenolic compounds which serve as germ and fungus-killing agents in such products as adhesives, paints, lacquers, paper coating, wood preservatives, shampoos, and laundry starches. Dioxin has caused cancer when given to animals. It primarily affects the liver and large intestine. Side effects are headaches, pain, excessive sweating, increased heart rates and respiratory difficulties.

Dioxin is a by-product of hexachlorophene, a compound that used to be used in toothpastes and as an antibacterial chemical in soaps, deodorants, and vaginal aerosol sprays. In 1972, seventy-two French infants were dusted with talc that had accidentally been mixed with 6 percent hexachlorophene. The infants all died. The FDA banned hexachlorophene, but not until millions of people had used it in all kinds of products. Hexachlorophene had been used since the 1940s and it was not until the early 1970s that repeated use of this drug led to significant amounts passing into the bloodstream. It accumulates in the blood. The ironic part is that this drug was shown to be ineffective. One of the investigations even showed that routine bathing of infants with hexachlorophene could result in an increase of staph infections.

Valium is the most over-prescribed drug and probably the most abused drug in the United States. It has shown to produce some of the symptoms it is supposed to relieve. Many women have died in hospital emergency rooms from the misuse of tranquilizers valium. How many deaths are attributed to an overdose of herbs?

DES (diethylstilbestrol) is a drug that was prescribed for women in the 1950s and 60s to help prevent miscarriage. Many children born of mothers who had taken the drug are now coming down with vaginal cancer and some of the girls have had to have their vaginas replaced. Of course, they will never be able to have children. The male offspring of mothers who took the drug were found to have genitourinary defects.

DES is a synthetic sex hormone discovered in 1938. It has been injected into the necks of chickens to make them grow faster. In 1947 the FDA authorized its use in poultry. It was known even back then that it caused cancer in animals, and possibly in humans.

In 1954 it was approved for cattle feed. It was believed not to be in the meat when it was slaughtered, but one year later the drug residue was found in the liver; kidney and skin fat of chickens, just before they were killed. It took four years after that before it was banned in poultry, but it still wasn't banned in cattle. It was still believed the residue was not in the cattle if they withdrew the drug 48 hours before they were slaughtered. Although it was banned in 1971 for pregnant women, the population was being drugged through the beef supply. Twenty-one other nations outlawed DES. Many countries, including Sweden, refused to import beef from the U.S. because of DES. However, there are also at least fourteen other hormones being fed to cattle.

THE STORY OF THALIDOMIDE

There are many drugs that have caused untold misery to thousands of people. One of the worst disasters in the field of medicine took place when I was pregnant with my youngest son in 1961. In the late 1950s, sleeping pills and tranquilizers were all the rage. Mothers in forty-six countries around the world, including thousands in the United States, gladly took a tranquilizing pill that was said to be safe and non-toxic for pregnant women. This wonder drug was thalidomide. Its most terrifying side effect was missing limbs on newborn infants. Fingers and ears were missing, and cleft palate was common. Some had paralyzed faces, brain damage, deafness, or blindness. The truth is that eight thousand babies were horribly poisoned and entered the world with terrible deformities. It is estimated that 16 thousand died at birth, mostly from internal damage. Many hundreds of other babies suffered from faulty hearts, hearing defects and other abnormalities that have not been attributed to thalidomide because they do not fit the most typical pattern. The sad story is told in a book called *Suffer The Children: The Story of Thalidomide.*

The anguish of the parents was aggravated by the fact that many did not know that thalidomide was to blame, since the pill had been prescribed months earlier to help them sleep, to relieve headaches, or to quiet morning sickness. Many parents believed that something must have been wrong with them and they blamed themselves or each other for the child's deformities. Thousands of people suffered with this supposedly innocent drug, developed and prescribed by modern medicine.

Experiences like these only reinforce my belief that the medical profession should be very humble when they say that herbs are dangerous. Of course, there are useful drugs, such as digitalis and penicillin. And there are times when a visit to the doctor is a wise choice; however, in most cases, the body will heal itself when given the correct diet, nutrients and herbs.

Amazingly, thalidomide has recently been approved by the World Health Organization to be used again. On March 5, 1996, Dr. Nancy Snyderman announced that the FDA was looking into approving thalidomide to use in patients with AIDS, cancer and TB. On May 13, 1994 a news documentary focused on how thalidomide was being used to treat leprosy in Brazil. There are an estimated million people in Brazil suffering from leprosy. One of the victims is a nine year-old without legs. The mother had taken thalidomide nine years ago. Another woman who had been on thalidomide for six years decided to have a child and her baby was born with no legs and arms. Another couple had a baby girl with short arms. One husband used the drug, gave it to his wife, and she had a son with no arms. Another woman got the drug from her sister and had a daughter who has shortened arms.

Undercover cameras discovered that the use of thalidomide is not controlled in Brazil and people can freely buy it. It was approved by the World Health Organization because it was easy to prescribe and inexpensive. Drug companies have responded to the relative freedom with irresponsibility. People are still being killed and maimed because in underdeveloped areas drug companies suppress information that they are compelled to make available in Britain and America.

8

COMMONLY USED HERBS

Herbs work in an natural way, unlike drugs, which can cause an array of side effects. Drugs often treat the *symptoms* of a disease and can create a feeling that all is well without getting to the real *cause* of the problem. Herbs, on the other hand, provide a complete and synergistic array of compounds designed by nature to increase the body's natural ability to heal itself. Herbs are less toxic than drugs and, when used wisely, can benefit and nourish the body.

There are some exceptional herbs that have been researched and found to be superior to drugs. Michael T. Murray, N.D., illustrates this by comparing a special licorice extract, DGL, that has been shown to be more effective than the drugs Zantac and Tagamet in comparison studies. The licorice extract shows no side effects and actually increases healing of the lining of the stomach while Zantac and Tagamet list side effects such as digestive disturbances, liver dysfunction, nutritional imbalances, and the return of ulcers after the drugs are stopped. Murray also compares the drug Proscar with serenoa extract (saw palmetto berry). Numerous studies have shown serenoa extract to be effective in nearly 90 percent of patients (Murray 1992, 88). The following herbs are some of the most common that have been extensively researched to be used in the place of drugs.

ASTRAGALUS (*Astragalus membranaceus*)

Traditional Chinese medicine has used astragalus for thousands of years for high blood pressure, viral infections, and immune system disorders. Recent studies have found that astragalus may be useful for cases of myasthenia gravis (Flynn, 4).

Astragalus helps increase the production of interferon, which helps stimulate and enhance the immune system. It is an excellent herb to protect against the increasing autoimmune diseases. Astragalus has been used to treat pneumonia, emphysema, chronic infection, chronic cough, uterine bleeding, chronic nephritis and ulcers. It will also help strengthen digestion, increase metabolism, low energy, and promote wound healing. No known toxicity has been found.

Complementary agents are echinacea, boneset, garlic, essential fatty acids, hawthorn, ginseng, schizandra, myrrh gum and prickly ash, ginkgo, suma, cat's claw, vitamin C with bioflavonoids, vitamins A and E, and selenium, and zinc. Chlorophyll and blue-green algae are beneficial.

BILBERRY (*Vaccinium myrtillus*)

Bilberry is an old remedy that has now been rediscovered. Research has found bilberry benefits the eyes because it strengthens the capillaries that surround them. It is a an antioxidant and will benefit the entire circulatory system, the brain, heart, feet, and hands. Bilberry inhibits blood platelets sticking together so blood clots can be reduced. Studies have found that bilberry extract can kill or inhibit the growth of certain fungi, yeast, and bacteria (Guinness, 324).

Used along with vitamin E and other supplements that supply oxygen to the blood, bilberry is considered and herb beneficial in preventing cataracts. It also has the ability to protect the eyes against damage caused by diabetes. Bilberry extracts in extensive studies in humans and animals have shown no toxic effects even when given at huge levels for long periods of time (Murray, 292).

Complementary agents are goldenseal, fenugreek, gimnema, vitamin C with biolfavonoids, ginkgo, bee polllen, L-carnitine, coenzyme Q_{10}, capsicum, germanium, suma, evening primrose oil, salmon oil, chlorophyll, lecithin, and free-form amino acids.

CAT'S CLAW (*Uncaria tomentosa*)

Cat's claw is known for its medicinal value throughout the Spanish-speaking world. It is also recognized as a valuable herb in Europe. Ongoing research seems to validate the usefulness of cat's claw. It is now gaining popularity in the United States as more people become familiar with the value of its multiple uses. Keplinger's research supports the use of cat's claw for immune system stimulation (Cerri, 257–61). Two compounds contained in this herb have also demonstrated the ability to inhibit the multiplication of some viruses (Aquino, 559–64). Doctors in Peru have successfully used the herb in treating fourteen types of diagnosed cancer (43).

Cat's claw has the ability to act as an antioxidant, protecting the body from free-radical damage and destroying or neutralizing carcinogens before they can damage the cells. It has been recognized that the herb helps support the body during chemotherapy and radiation and may even inhibit the growth of cancer cells. Cat's claw has also been used successfully to treat conditions associated with a weakened immune system such as AIDS, herpes, and Epstein-Barr syndrome. Its ability to strengthen the immune function really is remarkable. Other clinical research has found that cat's claw has the ability to reduce inflammation. It has also been used to help with allergies, hemorrhoids, ulcers, parasites, Crohn's disease, and gastrointestinal disorders. European studies have shown that cat's claw has extremely low toxicity, even when taken in large doses.

Complementary agents are pau d'arco, echinacea, glucosamine, cascara sagrada, acidophilus, shark cartilage, slippery elm, blue-green algae, vitamin A, B-complex, vitamin C with bioflavonoids, grape seed extract, essential fatty acids, and bee pollen.

ECHINACEA (*Echinacea purpurea*)

Echinacea contains natural antibiotic properties and is excellent for infections of all kinds. It stimulates the immune response by increasing the production of white blood cells and thus improving the body's ability to resist infections. The herb improves lymphatic filtration and drainage and helps remove toxins from the blood. It has cortisone-like properties that contribute to its anti-inflammatory action. Echinacea is

❖

recommended for stubborn viral infections, yeast infections, and arthritic conditions.

The ability of this herb to boost immune function deals with thymus gland stimulation (Gillum, 58). Echinacea has not exhibited any observed toxicity even in high doses. Used as an antibiotic herb for infections and cleansing the blood occasionally, it should not cause any problems.

Complementary agents are capsicum, astragalus, myrrh gum, prickly ash, licorice, chaparral, golden seal, garlic, burdock, cat's claw, vitamin C with bioflavonoids, vitamin A, blue-green algae, B-complex vitamins, calcium-magnesium, and zinc.

FEVERFEW (*Chrysanthemum parthenium*)

Feverfew has long been known and used in Europe as a natural remedy for pain relief and is considered an excellent remedy for severe headaches. In times past, feverfew was used just as aspirin and codeine are used today. This herb was used to treat any ailment where chills, fever, and headache developed.

Feverfew's active chemical, parthenolide, is similar to aspirin's acetyl-salicylic acid in that it inhibits prostaglandin production. It helps reduce inflammation and lessens pain in migraine headaches. It helps the body heal swelling, inflammation, and aches and pain (Hancock, xiv). Today, in Europe and now in the United States, feverfew is also known to be effective for migraine headaches, . It is good for relieving colds, dizziness, tinnitus, and inflammation from arthritis. Feverfew contains elements that work synergistically to regulate normal function of the body and allow the body to heal itself (Tenney, 80).

Feverfew has demonstrated few side effects. The side effects noticed have been mouth and throat irritation in allergic reaction (Hancock, xix). In two clinical trials, more side effects were reported by placebo groups than by feverfew groups (British Herbal Compendium, 97).

Complementary agents are white willow bark, passionflower, hops, scullcap, St. John's wort, kava, wood betony and valerian root. Vitamin C with bioflavonoids, vitamin A, E, selenium, and zinc are also good, as are lecithin, evening primrose oil, blue-green algae and salmon oil. External agents are tea tree oil and liquid minerals.

❖

GARLIC (*Allivum sativum*)

Garlic contains allicin and ajoene, which give the plant its natural antibiotic properties. It is effective against bacteria that may be resistant to other antibiotics, and it stimulates the lymphatic system to throw off waste materials. Garlic is a health-building and disease-preventing herb.

Controlled studies have discovered that garlic can lower cholesterol and triglyceride levels, reduce the tendency of the blood to clot, and decrease blood pressure (Guinness, 308). Dr. Erik Block discovered that garlic also protects the liver from drugs, radiation, and free radical damage (Weiner, 160). Garlic can be used for arthritis, asthma, blood poisoning, high or low blood pressure, bronchitis, cancer, candida, circulatory insufficiency, colds, colitis, coughs, digestive disorders, ear infections, fever, flu, fungus, gas, heart disease, infections (viral and bacterial), liver ailments, lung disorders, parasites, pinworm, prostate gland disorders and respiratory problems.

For colds, flu, and infections, mix 12 cloves of garlic, 1 cup of fresh lemon or lime juice, and 1 tablespoon pure honey in a blender. Take the mixture every half hour throughout the day. It is much safer than antibiotics and will not upset the natural flora. Garlic is considered safe, but an excess amount at one time could cause stomach upset.

Complementary agents are vitamin C with bioflavonoids, vitamin A, blue-green algae, chlorophyll, wheat grass juice, kelp, black walnut, red clover, goldenseal, echinacea, phytonutrients, cat's claw and bee pollen.

GINKGO (*Ginkgo biloba*)

Ginkgo is an adaptogen herb that helps the body deal with stressful situations. It increases oxygen and blood flow to the brain and extremities, improving mental clarity and inhibiting free radical scavengers from destroying cells. Ear and eye problems are also improved with ginkgo due to improved blood flow to nerves of the head. Ginkgo's ability to stimulate circulation and increase oxygen flow to neural tissue is impressive. This ability increases oxygen transport at the blood-brain barrier site while inhibiting the permeability of toxins into brain tissue (Hindmarch and Subhan, 89–93). In a double-blind study one group of healthy young women received ginkgo extract, and another was given a

✥

placebo. A memory test was administered and the reaction time in those women who had taken the ginkgo improved significantly. These findings corresponded with EEG tracings that showed increased brain wave activity (Gebner and Klasser, 1459–65).

Ginkgo can be beneficial for Alzheimer's disease, asthma, depression, attention deficit disorder, blood clots, circulatory insufficiency, dementia, kidney disease, memory loss, respiratory disease, senility, stress, stroke, tinnitus and vascular disease.

Ginkgo is considered nontoxic and virtually without side effects. In very rare cases, some gastric upset or incidence of headache or skin rash has occurred. The herb can be used with other supplements such as ginseng, sage, bee pollen, capsicum, suma, St. John's wort, garlic, vitamin B-complex, folic acid, magnesium, choline, lecithin, coenzyme Q_{10}, germanium, bilberry, milk thistle, and butcher's broom.

GOLDENSEAL (*Hydrastis canadensis*)

Goldenseal has natural antibiotic properties to stop infections and kill toxins, parasites, and worms in the body. This herb also has constituents that help improve and regulate liver function. It is a valuable herb for all catarrhal conditions, whether in the nasal area, bronchial tubes, throat, intestines, stomach, or bladder.

The bitter properties of goldenseal makes it an effective remedy for digestive disorders. Clinical studies have proven goldenseal's ability to protect against gram-positive and gram-negative bacteria, including tuberculosis bacteria. It helps to reduce vaginal and uterine inflammation. Tests have found that berberine-containing herbs such as goldenseal can be more effective in treating gastrointestinal infections than standard antibiotics (Elkins, 49).

Goldenseal is beneficial as an antibiotic and can be used for internal bleeding, eye infections, all other infections, excessive menstruation, vaginitis, colon inflammation, liver problems, mouth sores, worms and parasites, venereal disease, herpes, ringworm, and cancer.

Prolonged use of goldenseal is not recommended. Short periods for one week at a time is very beneficial and seems to cause no problems. Pregnant women should not use this herb as its berberine content could stimulate uterine contractions.

❖

Complementary agents are barberry, Oregon grape, echinacea, garlic, capsicum, myrrh, ginger, eyebright, juniper, dandelion, black cohosh, comfrey, cascara, gentian, dong quai, vitamin C with bioflavonoids, vitamin A, digestive enzymes, and grape seed.

HAWTHORN BERRY (*Crategus oxyacantha*)

Hawthorn is well known as a botanical heart tonic and is traditionally used to treat high and low blood pressure, irregular heartbeat, heart pain and atherosclerosis. This herb has been used in preventing arteriosclerosis and in helping such conditions as heart valve defects, an enlarged heart, angina pectoris, and difficult breathing due to ineffective heart action and lack of oxygen in the blood.

The cardiotonic properties of hawthorn have been shown to be effective in clinical studies. The flavonoid content of the herb has been shown to dilate peripheral and coronary blood vessels, which helps alleviate hypertension and angina (Flynn, 47). It is also worth noting that using the herb over long periods of time can escalate its benefits (Guinness, 311). One of the important benefits of hawthorn is its ability to lower serum cholesterol levels and prevent cholesterol deposits from accumulating in arteries (Murray, 383).

No known toxicity has been found in hawthorn. The effects of hawthorn can be cumulative. Complementary agents are capsicum, garlic, passionflower, hops, valerian, ginkgo, suma, parsley, ginseng, butcher's broom, kelp, skullcap, mistletoe, licorice, evening primrose oil, salmon oil, vitamin E, vitamin C with bioflavonoids, chlorophyll, and blue-green algae.

LICORICE (*Glycyrrhiza glabra*)

Licorice possesses antiarthritic and anti-inflammatory properties that make it effective for low adrenal function. Such stimulation helps counteract stress and supplies energy to the body. The Chinese regard licorice as a great detoxifier. It is often used in Chinese medicine and is believed to increase strength and endurance. It is also used to treat disorders such as female problems, fevers, infections and colds, and enhances the ability of other herbs.

The properties in licorice (glycyrrhizin and glycyrrhetinic acid) stimulate the production of interferon in the body, which helps protect the immune system. Scientific research has discovered that licorice contains anti-inflammatory properties, anti-allergic, and estrogenic action. Licorice may also be useful for protecting against and healing ulcers as well as a treatment for hepatitis. It is also being studied as a therapy for Addison's disease, which involves inadequate adrenal function (Tenney, 73).

Licorice is beneficial for adrenal exhaustion, drug withdrawal, colds, female complaints, hypoglycemia, expels phlegm, tonic, blood cleanser, cough, energy, hoarseness, lung problems, liver, circulation, endurance, impotency, ulcers. Persons low in potassium and minerals may have a rise in blood pressure. It should be monitored in those with high blood pressure.

Complementary agents are wild yam, saw palmetto, dong quai, black cohosh, kelp, gotu kola, milk thistle, dandelion, ginger, ginseng, queen of the meadow, sarsaparilla, cramp bark, squaw vine, bee pollen, chlorophyll, blue-green algae, parsley, bilberry, vitamin E, B-complex, folic acid, calcium/magnesium, and potassium.

MILK THISTLE (*Silybum marianum*)

Milk thistle is an excellent treatment for liver disease because it can block damage to and regenerate liver cells. It also acts as an antioxidant that protects against free-radical damage. A healthy liver will protect the immune system and protect against diseases. The liver is responsible for detoxifying the body. Anytime we ingest potentially harmful chemicals, which include drugs or alcohol, liver cells must filter out these toxins.

Experiments using silymarin from milk thistle show that when the herb was given before a deadly mushroom amanita toxin was ingested, it was 100 percent effective in preventing liver toxicity (Desplaces et al., 89–96). It can also help in gallbladder disease. Studies show that taking milk thistle helps to reduce cholesterol buildup in the bile (Murray, *The Healing Power of Herbs*, 244).

Milk thistle is beneficial for gallbladder, spleen, and stomach problems, liver damage, alcoholism, cirrhosis, skin problems, fatty deposits, heartburn, indigestion, appetite stimulant, protects against chemotherapy,

❖

depression, gas hepatitis, and radiation. There is no known toxicity. It may produce looser stools, although the effect is rare.

Complementary agents are dandelion, vitamin C with bioflavonoids, grape seed extract, pau d'arco, turmeric, artichoke, schisandra, suma, vitamin E, selenium, germanium, chlorophyll, blue-green algae, essential fatty acids, licorice, burdock, cascara sagrada, and psyllium.

PAU D' ARCO/TAHEEBO (*Tabebuia avellandedae*)

Pau d'arco has powerful antibiotic and virus-killing properties. Its compounds seem to attack the very cause of disease. It acts as a blood tonic and helps the proper assimilation of nutrients and the elimination of wastes. It's anti-inflammatory properties help reduce pain.

It helps to strengthen the liver and remove poisons from liver tissue. It's high iron content boosts the assimilation of vital nutrients. It works as a natural antibiotic, antiviral, antibacterial, and antifungal agent. It is an excellent protection for the entire body. Scientific studies done in the 1970s and 1980s show that lapachol, the key component of pau d'arco, is effective against viral infections, parasites, and cancers of all kind (Tenney, *Encyclopedia,* 80). Pau d'arco is also beneficial for AIDS, blood disorders, candida, infections, liver disease, pain, prostate disorders, ringworm, ulcers, anemia, cancer, diabetes, herpes, hypoglycemia, lupus, parasites, skin diseases, tumors, venereal disease, and yeast infections.

Using the whole herb in tea form is recommended and generally considered safe. If nausea occurs, it may be the liver trying to detoxify.

Complementary agents are licorice, garlic, echinacea, burdock, goldenseal, black walnut, alfalfa, kelp, milk thistle, dandelion, Oregon grape, yellow dock, yerba santa, vitamin E, vitamin C with bioflavonoids, beta carotene, natural sodium, potassium, calcium and magnesium, chlorophyll, blue-green algae, and essential fatty acids.

ST. JOHN'S WORT (*Hypericum perforatum*)

St. John's wort is an herb used for anxiety and depression. Recent research has found that a key component of the herb, hypericin, has the ability to alter brain chemistry. Clinical studies show that St. John's wort is useful for treating depression and alleviating anxiety and feelings of

❖

worthlessness (Murray, 226). St. John's wort is also beneficial for antiviral therapy, afterpains, skin problems, AIDS, cancer therapy, bronchitis, insomnia, nervousness, tumors, blood purifier, hysteria, melancholy, and spasms.

There are no significant side effects associated with using St. John's wort extract. Complementary agents are ginger, capsicum, lady's slipper, scullcap, hops, evening primrose oil, borage, black currant, flaxseed oil, burdock, vitamin B-complex, vitamin B_6 and vitamin B_{12} (sublingual), folic acid, calcium/magnesium, wild yam, and digestive enzymes.

SAW PALMETTO (*Serenoa repens*)

Saw palmetto has been used to treat conditions of the genito-urinary system. It acts as an antiseptic, reduces excessive mucus in the head and sinuses, and is used for both male and female reproductive organs. Clinical studies have discovered that saw palmetto is beneficial in treating prostate problems. In fact, it has been proven to work better than the pharmaceutical drug Proscar for enlarged prostate glands (Braeckman, 776–85). Saw palmetto may be beneficial for women who suffer from hormonal imbalances by helping to normalize estrogen levels. It is also used in digestive formulas because of its ability to stimulate normal appetite and boost nutrient assimilation (Elkins, 75).

Saw palmetto is used to treat the following: hormone regulation, impotency, prostate, reproductive organs, genitourinary problems, infertility, bronchitis, colds, menstrual disorders, ovarian dysfunction, lactation, thyroid deficiencies, digestive problems, painful periods. There is no known toxicity when using saw palmetto.

Complementary agents are ginseng, sarsaparilla, suma, bee pollen, fennel, catnip, capsicum, ginger, echinacea, pau d'arco, uva ursi, kelp, marshmallow, B-complex vitamins, beta carotene, calcium/magnesium, zinc, selenium, digestive enzymes, essential fatty acids, and pumpkin seeds.

SUMA (*Pfaffia paniculata*)

Suma is adaptogen herb rich in nutrients that help protect the immune system, relieve stress, and help the body adapt to environmental and psychological stresses. It is an herb beneficial for both men and women because of its ability to restore sexual function and to protect against viral infections. Another benefit of this herb is that it contains two plant hormones, sitosterol and stipmasterol, found to be beneficial to human metabolism by increasing circulation and decreasing high blood cholesterol levels.

The Portuguese call suma "para todo," meaning *for everything*—a good indication of all this herb is capable of. Suma has been used traditionally to strengthen the immune system and to treat immune related diseases such as cancer, leukemia, Hodgkin's diseases, and diabetes. It enhances energy in the body and promotes longevity. It also relieves stress, protects against viral infections, restores sexual function, lowers cholesterol, improves circulation, and helps with degenerative diseases, fatigue, hormone imbalances, and immune system disorders.

There is no record of toxicity when using suma. Complementary agents are ginkgo, ginseng, bee pollen, royal jelly, echinacea, astragalus, kelp, licorice, burdock, schizandra, ginger, capsicum, garlic, blue-green algae, chlorophyll, germanium, coenzyme Q_{10}, vitamins A, C, and E, and selenium and zinc. B-complex vitamins, digestive enzymes, hydrochloric acid are also excellent to supplement.

VALERIAN (*Valeriana officinalis*)

Studies have identified one of the most valuable properties of valerian as its ability to produce a deep, satisfying sleep. The herb acts as a relaxant and is an effective remedy for insomnia (D. Tenney, 10). Valerian works similar to other standard sleep aids often prescribed, but its advantage lies in the fact that it does not cause the morning grogginess often associated with prescription sleep drugs (*Valerian*, 325).

Besides being beneficial for insomnia, valerian also helps with anxiety and stress. It is useful for all kinds of sleep disorders, especially when they are related to anxiety, nervousness, headache pain, or physical or mental exhaustion. It is used for hypertension, heart disorders, afterbirth pains, anxiety, tension, high blood pressure, stress, nervous stomach, palpitations, menstrual cramps, and muscle spasms.

No known toxicity exists. Extreme doses should be avoided, and one should alternate valerian with other nervine herbs such as hops, skullcap,

❖

St. John's wort, catnip, lady's slipper, chamomile, kava kava, and passionflower. Complementary agents are hops, chamomile, passionflower, scullcap, wood betony, black cohosh, calcium/magnesium, B-complex vitamins, and niacin.

VITEX (*Vitex agnus-castus*)

Vitex is considered a very beneficial herb for women's ailments. Scientific research has shown that the extract has the ability to help restore normal ovulation and menstrual cycles. It strengthens the pituitary to release hormones that balance estrogen and progesterone, mainly boosting the progesterone levels.

Vitex, like many other herbs, especially demonstrates its benefits after a few months of use. Besides strengthening the female organs, vitex helps with water retention, emotional upsets, migraine headaches, mastitis, and menstrual cramps. As far as fertility, it may be beneficial in regulating the ovulatory cycle. In menopause it can help with hot flashes, depression, and dry vagina.

Vitex has an excellent safety record. There have been no reports of side effects in the over 2,000 years it has been used. Complementary agents are dong quai, black cohosh, wild yam, cramp bark, saw palmetto, prickly ash, evening primrose oil, vitamin E, calcium/magnesium, B-complex vitamins, blue-green algae, chlorophyll, digestive enzymes and free-form amino acids.

9

METAL POISONING:
A HEALTH HAZARD

TOXIC METALS

Toxic metals are systemic poisons that inhibit biochemical enzyme functioning and can cause fatigue from body malfunction. These toxic metals are non-essential trace metals, and they are known to accumulate in the tissues and biological fluids, producing acute and chronic toxicity.

Depression and suicidal thoughts seem to be a natural part of heavy metal poisoning. Mental depression has a sudden onset and usually is not caused by any one set of circumstances. It seems to arrive when everything is going great. Doctors (after putting their depressed patients through numerous tests) finally refer them to a psychiatrist, which only prolongs their misery. This can make them feel guilty for the feelings they can't control.

Common toxic metals are aluminum, arsenic, cadmium, lead, mercury, and nickel. Nickel is widely used as a catalyst to harden fats. It is found in most margarines, commercial peanut butter, and hardened shortening. It is in drinking water, refined and processed foods, superphosphate fertilizers, and tobacco smoke.

ALUMINUM

Aluminum contamination is a major health threat today. High levels are showing up in the human body. Absorption of aluminum by the body is not only associated with Alzheimer's disease, but also with Parkinson's disease and dialysis dementia. It also lowers the body's immune system. Pots and pans, foil, antacids, and baking powder are common items with aluminum. It is found in pickles, relishes, and some cheeses, in soft drinks and beers in uncoated aluminum cans. It is also found in water supplies and the soil. Aluminum inhibits fluorine and phosphorus metabolism, resulting over a long period of time in a loss of essential minerals from the bones and sets the stage for osteoporosis. *The Harvard Medical School Newsletter* published an article that stated America is experiencing an epidemic of osteoporosis in the elderly and by the age of thirty-five the seed is sown.

ARSENIC

Arsenic is in our environment as a by-product of industry. It's in the air, a pollutant that we are exposed to each day of our lives. It is found in the refining process of glass making, pesticide plants spray, and in coal fired boilers. Arsenic is in coal and in the air wherever it is burned. Coal workers are at potential risk. It is also in hidden items such as dishwasher sealant and has been known to poison whole families. There is also an accumulation of arsenic from liquor.

Arsenic settles in the muscles and back. Spasms in the back can pull the spine out of place. Arsenic poisoning produces nervous irritations in various parts of the body. It is found mainly in the liver. In females arsenic levels increase in the blood during menstruation and during the fifth and sixth months of pregnancy. Symptoms of arsenic toxicity are fatigue, loss of pain sensation, and inflammation of the lining membrane of the stomach and intestines (gastroenteritis). Arsenic replaces essential trace minerals, which disrupts the body's metabolism.

CADMIUM

Cadmium is a by-product of industry and is extremely widespread. It is in the air, soil, and water. It is used as a hardener in tires. We acquire it by absorbing it through our tissues. People with hypertension usually have elevated cadmium levels and are usually low in zinc. It affects the pancreas and spleen. Coronary disease tends to rise when the intake of cadmium is high. It is also found in bone marrow and in the male testes.

Cadmium can produce high blood pressure, kidney and liver damage, anemia, and a host of other symptoms as well as fatigue. Scientists used to think that nothing could remove cadmium deposits. Science has since proven that iron and vitamin C together can reduce cadmium levels. Selenium and zinc are the best protection against cadmium toxicity.

LEAD

Lead poisoning, as we have mentioned before, is a major pollutant in our environment, and we breathe it constantly. It is a frightening health threat to our children. Lead causes a gradual buildup of chronic problems, such as allergies. It also decreases immunity to diseases. It accumulates in the tissues. Low levels can bring subtle changes and problems. It is felt that most people in the United States may be suffering partial brain dysfunction as a result of lead pollution. Lead intake increases 25 percent when you smoke.

Lead deposits in the brain and causes brain damage, retardation, and hyperactivity. Many children are born with high levels of lead and cadmium, which causes nervous disorders similar to epileptic-type nerve transmission problems. When lead goes into the brain, it displaces copper, iron, and zinc. Oxygen is essential to proper brain function, and the lack of copper in the brain causes the cells to "breathe" with difficulty. Zinc deficiency can cause learning and memory difficulties.

Lead interferes with the normal activities of the nervous system and causes damage to the myelin sheath (a fat-like substance forming the principal component in the brain and the covering over the nerves).

Lead interferes with the energy in the body, with enzyme exchange, as well as with the nervous system. It accumulates in the bones and displaces calcium. It causes the body to be more susceptible to diseases, muscle weakness, tremors, gout, lack of coordination, clumsiness, and symptoms similar to multiple sclerosis.

Lead by-products are found in auto exhaust, air pollution, canned food and canned drinks, mascara, pewter tableware, plumbing, roadside vegetables, tobacco smoke, water, wine, some hair colorings, and ceramic glaze. Lead activates the enzyme hyaluronidase, which breaks down the synovial fluid in bone joints. It also contributes to the deterioration of tissue and collagen and makes people more susceptible to diseases like cancer and arthritis.

MERCURY

The amalgam used to fill teeth is 40 to 50 percent mercury. Under the pressure of hard chewing, mercury vapor is released from the fillings and is absorbed by the body. To make matters worse, the bacteria in the mouth (the same strain blamed for plaque) can convert mercury into methyl mercury, the most toxic form. It is not only toxic, but has an affinity for proteins, attaching itself to blood cells and interfering with the function of the glands, nervous system, and the brain. It has a potentially dangerous effect on the lungs, heart, liver, and kidneys.

It depresses the immune system. Dr. Carlton Fredericks said that mercury toxicity could have been responsible for some of his patients' susceptibility to yeast infections and allergies.

Mercury is found in treated seeds for farm planting, cosmetics, fabric softeners, fish and sea foods, fungicides, laxatives containing calomel, and some hemorrhoidal suppository preparations.

Mercury causes depression, irritability, tremors, dizziness, and diarrhea. As the metal builds up over a period of years, it leads to progressive degeneration of the brain, liver, kidneys, and intestines.

NICKEL

Nickel settles in the sinuses, head, heart, or spinal column. It acts as a poison to the nervous system. Too much nickel in the human body may paralyze the spinal column. Many locked joints are caused by an accumulation of nickel. It is cancer-causing, and respiratory cancer has been known to develop within three years of inhaling nickel-contaminated dust. Nickel carbonyl is found in cigarette smoke and is harmful to both the smoker and non-smoker who breath "second-hand" cigarette smoke pollution.

❖

PROTECTION AGAINST TOXIC METALS

Vitamin A is necessary for the cells to be able to eliminate the toxic metal absorbed from chemicals in food, air, and water.

Vitamin B-complex protects the immune system. Under stress the B vitamins need to be increased. They protect the nerve sheath and prevent lead from damaging the nervous system.

Vitamin C with bioflavonoids stimulates natural interferon production in the body. Interferon protects and strengthens the immune system. Vitamin C is essential to take each day to keep our tissues saturated and protect the body from toxic metals. Bioflavonoids increase the strength of the capillary walls, reduce inflammation, and help keep the collagen healthy. Collagen is a cement that sticks the cells together and is essential for healthy muscles, skin, and joints.

Fiber dilutes stool bile acids and reduces the concentration of toxic carcinogenic substances in the colon and eliminates them. Fiber also eliminates excess fat in the body. Fiber such as psyllium, oat bran, and whole grains are excellent. Apple pectin removes lead. It is changed into galacturonic acid (one of nature's cleansing agents) after digestion. This acid combines with lead to form an insoluble metallic salt that cannot be absorbed. Eat fiber daily.

Oral chelation is a formula with vitamins, minerals, glandulars, amino acids, and herbs used to clean the system. They are natural nutrients that gradually dissolve and eliminate deposits on the arteries. It is very effective to rid the body of high levels of toxic metals.

Distilled water is a natural chelation. Always use with minerals.

Lecithin combines with choline and produces acetylcholine, a vital neurotransmitter. Lecithin is an essential brain food.

Calcium is an indispensable mineral; it actually penetrates the bones and slowly displaces lead. It prevents accumulation of lead from the intestinal tract. The best calcium is an herbal calcium formula.

Germanium binds with toxic metals to prevent them from being dispersed throughout the body. It improves stamina and endurance. It increases the body's production of interferon, which stops the multiplication of viruses.

Garlic is a natural antibiotic, lowers blood pressure, cleans the veins, helps in digestion, and is excellent for lungs and respiratory problems.

❖

Garlic is rich in sulphur, which attracts metals and eliminates them from the body. Garlic contains germanium and selenium with chelation ability to neutralize heavy metal toxicity.

Ginkgo is a strong antioxidant, free-radical scavenger, and increases the flow of nutrients and oxygen to all cells. It improves memory, mental efficiency, and concentration, reduces anxiety, tension, symptoms of senility and age related cerebral disorders.

Gotu kola is food for the brain. It purifies the blood and helps eliminate fatigue and memory loss. It works to increase mental alertness and is a tonic for the whole body. The herb helps rebuild energy reserves, especially after a nervous breakdown, and protects the body against toxins.

Herbs containing sulphur are excellent to protect the body from heavy metal toxicity: horseradish, watercress, alfalfa, burdock, dandelion, comfrey, garlic, onions, sarsaparilla, kelp, echinacea, lobelia, mullein, parsley, cayenne, chaparral, eyebright, nettle, and fennel.

Zinc is an essential mineral and helps to eliminate lead from the body as well as other toxins.

Kelp attaches itself to any lead that is present and carries it harmlessly out of the system.

Coenzyme Q₁₀ protects the immune system, strengthens the body's resistance to stress and disease by making tissues stronger and healthier, aids in oxygenation within the cells and tissues. It is good for heart disease, aging, cancer, and obesity.

Chlorophyll is nature's natural cleanser. It cleans the blood stream and eliminates toxins from the bowels.

Suma contains germanium to protect the immune system. It protects the body from stress, improves circulation, and arthritis. It also balances hormones.

Algin is a natural extract from kelp. It is a concentrated form of nutrient that is very effective in eliminating radioactive strontium 90 from the body. It is also beneficial in eliminating the chemical additives that we ingest daily. Algin grabs hold of the toxic material and excretes it out of the body. It acts like a magnet, drawing the radioactive material and other unwanted toxic waste that is harmful to the system.

Nervine herbs are essential to protect the central nervous system and the

❖

brain. Good nervine herbs are hops, lady's slipper, skullcap, valerian, passionflower, wood betony, chamomile, black cohosh, and lobelia.

Hydrochloric acid and digestive enzymes are essential nutrients, binding metals and eliminating them from the body.

Selenium rids the body of lead, cadmium, mercury herbicides, pesticides and drugs.

10

MENUS AND RECIPES

Raw Food Diet
Liquids should be taken at least thirty minutes before meals.

Day One

Breakfast
Fresh sliced peaches, strawberries
    and bananas with nut milk
Fresh fruit juice

Lunch
Meatless loaf
Raw vegetable juice

Dinner
Sprout salad
Herbed yogurt dressing
Raw carrot juice

Day Two

Breakfast
Fruit sherbert with shredded
    fresh coconut

Lunch
Multi-seed loaf
Fresh vegetable juice

Dinner
Supper salad
Raw vegetable juice

Day Three

Breakfast
Nature's Cale
Herb tea

Lunch
Lentil soup
Raw vegetable juice

Dinner
Total Salad
Raw vegetable juice

Day Four

Breakfast
Apple Delight
Raw fruit juice

Lunch
Guacamole salad dip
Carrot sticks, celery sticks, cauli-
    flowerettes
Raw vegetable juice

Dinner
Stuffed peppers
Raw vegetable juice

Day Five

Breakfast
Banana Freeze
Fresh orange juice

Lunch
Cucumber salad
Raw vegetable juice

Dinner
Corned salad
Raw vegetable soup
Raw vegetable juice

Day Six

Breakfast
Gold salad
Raw fruit juice

Lunch
Green soup
Raw vegetable juice

Dinner
Veggie-fish loaf
Raw vegetable juice

Day Seven

Breakfast
Apples Plus
Fresh fruit juice

Lunch
Cabbage salad
Fresh vegetable juice

Dinner
Fiber loaf
Fresh vegetable juice

❖

RAW FOOD RECIPES

MEATLESS LOAF

1 c. grated carrots
1 c. diced tomatoes
1 c. chopped celery
1/4 c. diced green bell pepper
2 t. salad oils
1 c. ground almonds (or enough to make a firm loaf)
Pat into oiled dish and garnish with parsley.

FRUIT SHERBET

Blend orange juice, pineapple juice and diced fresh oranges and pineapple, plus one sliced banana in blender. Freeze in ice cube tray. Take frozen pieces and blend with lecithin granules, 4 T. honey, and a dash of cinnamon.

MULTI-SEED LOAF

Soak the seeds for eight hours; drain. Grind in blender:
1 c. sunflower seeds
1 c. sesame seeds
1 c. shredded raw potato
Mix with
1 c. shredded carrots
1 c. diced celery
1/2 c. chopped onion
1 c. diced tomato
Add enough tomato juice to moisten and mold into a loaf.

SUPPER SALAD

Dressing: plain yogurt, paprika, ground dill
2 Jerusalem artichokes, sliced thinly
2 T. chopped green onion
Dash of kelp
Red onion, separated into rings

1 small bunch of radishes, sliced
watercress, rinsed and chopped
torn salad greens (red leaf, beet greens)
1 sliced avocado
1 med. sliced tomato
1/2 cucumber, sliced
1 small green pepper, chopped
Lightly toss all vegetables together. Serve with dressing.

NATURE'S CAKE

1 c. rolled oats
1 c. ground almonds
1 t. cinnamon
1/2 t. nutmeg
1/4 t. cloves
1/2 c. unsweetened shredded coconut
1/4 c. honey
3 T. apple juice
3 T. raw applesauce
1/2 c. tahini (almond paste)
1 c. raisins
1/2 c. ground dates
3 c. shredded carrots
Grind the raisins, dates and carrots together and add to honey, apple juice and applesauce. Mix in tahini and dry ingredients. Pat into a loaf pan and refrigerate at least 2 hours.

LENTIL SOUP

2 c. sprouted lentils
1 med. potato, chopped
1/2 c. chopped parsley
1/2 c. chopped celery
2 c. grated zucchini
1/4 c. chopped onion
Blend. Heat and serve with dollop of plain yogurt.

TOTAL SALAD

1 c. mung bean sprouts
1 c. alfalfa sprouts
1/2 avocado, sliced
1 tomato, sliced
1 cucumber, sliced
radishes, sliced
1/2 c. sliced zucchini
1 small sliced bell pepper
1/2 c. sliced green onions
Mixed salad (dark) greens
Toss all together. Squeeze fresh lemon over salad and serve. Garnish with sunflower seeds.

APPLE DELIGHT

2 large apples, grated
1/4 c. raisins, ground
1/4 c. dates, ground
1/2 c. sunflower seeds, ground
1/2 c. apple juice
dash cinnamon
1 T. honey
Mix together, chill and serve.

GUACAMOLE

2 medium avocados, mashed
1 large peeled tomato, chopped
1 T. red minced onion
1 T. fresh parsley
1 T. fresh lemon juice
Kelp to taste
Mix all ingredients together and serve on a bed of fresh greens. Use as a dip with fresh vegetables.

STUFFED PEPPERS

2 large green peppers, cut in half
Mix together:
1/2 c. celery, chopped
1 tomato, chopped
3 green onions, chopped
1 c. fresh peas
1/4 c. ground almonds
homemade mayonnaise to moisten
Prepare green peppers and chill in cold water for a few hours. Mix all other ingredients together and fill the green pepper halves when ready to eat.

BANANA FREEZE

Blend 3 bananas in blender, with 1 t. fresh lemon juice, 1/4 t. cardamon, and 2 T. honey. Freeze in ice cube trays. Can be eaten fresh without freezing.

COOL SALAD

1 large sliced cucumber
3 large tomatoes, chopped
1 red pepper, chopped
1 c. mung bean sprouts
1/4 c. chopped raw cashews
1/4 lemon, juiced
2 T. chopped green onion
Vegetable seasoning to taste.
Mix all the ingredients in a large bowl.

RAW CARROT SOUP

1 c. carrot juice
1/2 lemon, juiced
1 t. olive oil
1 clove garlic
Blend, then mix in the following:
1/2 c. chopped tomato

1 t. chopped onion
1/2 c. grated celery
1/4 c. chopped red bell pepper

Corned Salad

4 ears sweet corn, scraped
1 c. diced, ripe tomato
1 c. shredded yellow crookneck squash
2 T. chopped green onion
2 T. chopped bell pepper
1/4 t. dill
1/4 t. marjoram
1/4 t. paprika
1 c. alfalfa sprouts
Mix together and serve with favorite dressing.

Gold Salad

1/2 c. soaked dried apricots
1 T. shredded fresh coconut
1 c. red seedless grapes
1 sliced banana
1 chopped ripe pear
2 T. almonds
Mix together and serve.

Green Soup

1 bunch green onions, chopped
1 c. shredded savoy cabbage
1 avocado
4 c. water
1 t. vegetable seasoning
1/4 t. cayenne pepper
Blend all vegetables, gradually adding 4 cups of water. Add vegetable seasonings and cayenne pepper.

VEGETABLE LOAF

1/2 c. chopped almonds
1 c. carrot pulp
2 stalks celery
1 c. chopped green onions
Fresh or dried basil
1/8 c. rejuvelac or water
1 c. sesame seeds
1/4 bunch finely chopped parsley
1 green pepper, minced
dill weed to taste
vegetable seasoning to taste
Grind almonds and seeds and add carrots, parsley, and remaining ingredients. Mix with hands. If too thick, add more water, a little at a time. Place in a dish and refrigerate for 6–8 hours.

APPLES PLUS

Six apples
2 bananas, diced
3 peaches, diced
2 pears, diced
Dig out the centers of apples, about 3/4 of way down. Add the apple pulp to rest of fruit, minus the seeds, core and membranes. Fill the apples with fruit stuffing and sprinkle with grated almonds.

CABBAGE SALAD

1 c. red cabbage, chopped
1 c. savoy cabbage, chopped
1/2 c. chopped celery
1 c. chopped red onion
1 c. coarsely chopped pecans
Leaf lettuce
Olive oil
Lemon juice
Mix and add equal parts olive oil and lemon juice. Serve on lettuce leaves.

❖

FIBER LOAF

2 c. ground sesame seeds
4 c. ground sunflower seeds
10 large mushrooms, chopped
1 c. diced parsley
3 cloves garlic, finely chopped
4 stalks celery, finely diced
pinch of sweet basil
1/2 tsp. dill
Vegetable seasoning to taste

Mix ground seeds together. Add enough water so that the ground seeds stick together. Add diced vegetables and seasonings, according to taste. Place in warm place 12-24 hours (70 degrees to 90 degrees) until top is firm.

Cooked Food Diet

Day One

Breakfast
Fruit salad
Steamed millet
(thermos method)

Lunch
Wild rice medley
Cheese enchiladas
Green salad

Dinner
Yam bake
Soup of the day

Day Two

Breakfast
Apple salad

Lunch
Steamed broccoli
Baked potato with yogurt
Green onions
Whole grain roll

Dinner
Vegetable chop suey
Steamed brown rice
Green salad

Day Three

Breakfast
Super breakfast cereal
Juice

Lunch
Pinto bean stew
Green salad

Dinner
Strawberry Jello salad

Day Four

Breakfast
Glazed fresh fruit
Steamed whole oats

Lunch
Spanish millet loaf
Whole grain roll

Dinner
Potato salad
Green salad

Day Five

Breakfast
Steamed wheat berries (thermos
    method)
Sliced peaches

Lunch
Lima bean casserole
Chapatis
Vegetable juice

Dinner
Barley salad
Whole grain roll

Day Six

Breakfast
Nut and seed granola
Sliced fruit in season

Lunch
Spaghetti squash with tomato
    squash and Italian seasoning
Steamed brown rice

Dinner
Navy bean soup
Whole grain roll
Vegetable juice

Day Seven

Breakfast
Fresh, sliced fruit in season with
    yogurt dressing

Lunch
Rice, Mexican style
Vegetable juice

Dinner
Summer salad

❖

COOKED FOOD RECIPES

WILD RICE MEDLEY

1/2 c. wild rice
1/2 c. Basmate rice
1/4 c. olive oil
1/2 onion, chopped
1/2 green pepper, chopped
1/4 c. chopped almonds
2 T. lemon juice

Heat 3 cups water to boiling. Add rice. Cook (covered) for 30 minutes. Turn off heat. Let pan sit for 20 minutes with lid on. This will finish steam cooking it. Toss with rest of ingredients. Add seasonings to taste.

CHEESE ENCHILADAS

12 corn tortillas
1 c. mild cheese, grated
1/2 c. onion, chopped
1 small can diced green chiles
1 large can enchilada sauce
1 small can tomato sauce
1 pint sour cream or mock sour cream
Black olives (optional) to sprinkle on top

Heat enchilada sauce and tomato sauce and add 1 small can of water. Mix the cheese, onions and chiles. Dip tortilla in the hot sauce mix to soften. Place about 2 T. of the cheese mixture on tortilla; top with a heaping tablespoon of sour cream; roll the tortilla and place seam side down and put in a baking dish. When all tortillas are rolled up, pour the rest of the enchilada sauce on the top and sprinkle top with cheese and olives. Bake at 350° for about 30 minutes.

Yam Bake

2 c. mashed, cooked yams or sweet potatoes
1 c. ripe mashed banana
1/3 c. yogurt or sour cream
1 egg
1/2 t. mineral salt
2 T. pure maple syrup or honey
Blend all ingredients together. Beat until smooth. Bake in a buttered casserole dish at 350° for 20 minutes. Serves 4–6.

Soup of the Day

Bring to boil:
2 quarts water
1 t. salt
1 t. garlic powder
2 t. chopped basil
2 small cans tomato sauce
Turn down heat and add sliced carrots, celery, cooked whole grain (rice or millet) in any quantity you desire. Simmer for 20 minutes.

Apple Salad

3 apples, cored and chopped
2 stalks celery, chopped
1 cup walnuts, chopped
Add salad dressing to moisten. Toss all ingredients together. Chill and serve.

Vegetable Chop Suey

1 c. green and red peppers, sliced diagonally
1 c. celery, sliced diagonally
1/2 c. onions, sliced
1 small can water chestnuts, sliced
1 c. bamboo shoots
1 c. mung bean sprouts
1 c. mushrooms, sliced

1/8 t. ginger
2 cloves garlic, minced
4 T. butter
4 t. tamari (soy sauce)
1 T. sesame seeds
Cook vegetables lightly and serve over cooked brown rice or millet. Vegetables should be crunchy.

SUPER BREAKFAST CEREAL

1/2 c. oatmeal
1 c. plain yogurt
1 T. orange juice
1 T. honey
1/2 c. raisins
1/4 c. almonds, chopped
1 T. sesame seeds
1/2 c. chopped peaches
1/2 c. chopped apples
1/2 c. sliced bananas
Mix all ingredients together. You can substitute sunflower seeds for sesame seeds and pecans for almonds.

STRAWBERRY JELL SALAD

I c. fruit and berry juice (frozen)
3 T. agar-agar flakes
3 T. honey
2 c. strawberries, sliced
2 bananas, sliced
1 T. fresh lemon juice
Dissolve agar-agar in the juice by bringing to a boil and simmer on low for about 5 minutes. Cool, add the strawberries, bananas, honey and lemon juice. Chill in a mold. Serves 6.

Pinto Bean Stew

2 c. pinto beans, cooked
4 c. vegetable broth
1 c. carrots, sliced
1/2 c. broccoli, sliced
1/2 c. zucchini
1/2 c. celery, sliced
3 large tomatoes, peeled and chopped
2 T. olive oil
1 T. vegetable seasoning
1 T. kelp

In a large stew pan, saute onions and garlic in oil. Add all ingredients and water if needed. Bring to a boil, reduce heat and simmer about 15 minutes, remove from heat while vegetables are still crunchy.

Glazed Fresh Fruit

1 c. fruit and berry juice, unsweetened (frozen section)
1 T. arrowroot or cornstarch
1/4 t. ginger
1/2 t. cardamon
2 c. fresh strawberries
1 c. apples, chopped
1 c. seedless grapes, halved
1 c. fresh peaches, sliced

Stir arrowroot and seasonings in juice over stove and bring to a boil; cook for one minute. Toss fruit together and fold in juice mixture and stir to coat well. Chill.

Spanish Millet Loaf

2 c. cooked millet
1 c. whole wheat bread crumbs
1 small can green chiles
1 c. canned tomatoes
2 beaten eggs
2 T. vegetable seasoning

1 c. ground almonds
2 T. olive oil
1 t. chili powder
Combine all ingredients together. Pour into a buttered loaf pan. Cook at at 350° for 45 minutes. While cooking, baste with butter two or three times. It may be served with uncooked salsa.

POTATO SOUP

4 large potatoes
3 c. water
2 T. raw cashew butter
1 small onion
4 stalks celery, chopped
1/2 c. freshly chopped parsley
1 t. vegetable salt
Steam potatoes with skins on in the water. Remove skin from potatoes and mash through dicer. Dissolve nut butter in 1 c. of warm purified water. Mix all other ingredients together and cook in double boiler for about 20 minutes.

LIMA BEAN CASSEROLE

4 c. cooked, fresh lima beans
1 c. finely chopped onions
2 cloves garlic, minced
1/2 t. kelp
1 grated carrot
2 stalks chopped celery
1 T. chopped red or green pepper
1 t. Italian mixed herbs
2 T. tomato paste
1 T. butter or olive oil
Put beans in a baking dish. Add all ingredients except juice and butter. Stir well. Add tomato paste and mix with beans. Pour melted butter or olive oil over top. Bake at 350° for 1 hour. Serves 6–8.

CHAPATIS

1 1/2 c. whole wheat pastry flour
1/2 c. waterÑmore if needed
1 T. cold pressed oil

Mix the flour, water and oil. Knead the dough until it is smooth and elastic. Pinch off the dough into balls. Should make about eight. Flatten the dough in the palm of your hand and roll it out on a floured surface into a circle about seven inches in diameter. Use an iron or stainless heavy griddle. Cook each side until brown. The pan needs to be hot enough or it will dry out. Clean burned flour from pan before cooking another.

BARLEY SALAD (AND SALAD DRESSING)

1 2/3 c. vegetable broth
1 c. whole barley, rinsed
1 c. grated carrots
1/2 c. sliced radishes
1/4 c. chopped fresh parsley
1 1/3 c. water
1/2 c. chopped green pepper
1/2 c. chopped red pepper
1/2 c. chopped Bermuda onion
1 T. dried dillweed

Bring water and broth to a boil, then add barley. Reduce heat, cover pan and simmer the barley for about an hour, or until done. Add cooked barley to dressing while it is still warm. Mix all ingredients well except the vegetables, which you can add and toss well just before serving.

Salad Dressing
1 pressed clove of garlic
1/2 t. vegetable seasoning
1/4 t. white pepper
2 T. olive oil
3 T. fresh lemon juice

Mix all dressing ingredients in a bowl.

Nut and Seed Granola

1 c. ground sunflower seeds
1 c. ground sesame seeds
1/8 c. ground chia seeds
1/8 c. ground flax seeds
1 c. freshly grated coconut
1 c. ground almonds
1 1/2 t. grated orange rind
1/2 t. cardamon
1/2 c. date sugar
1/2 c. warm honey
Mix all ingredients together and drip warm honey on them and stir. Keep in a tightly sealed jar in a cool place. Can cook in the oven at 200° for about an hour, stirring often.

Navy Bean Soup

2 c. navy beans
8 c. vegetable broth
1 c. sliced carrots
2 stalks celery, chopped
1 onion, minced
2 t. salt
Dash of herbs of choice (basil, mixed Italian, etc.)
Wash beans and soak in water overnight. Add soaked beans to boiling vegetable broth. Reduce heat and cook on low for an hour or until done. Add vegetables and herbs and cook for about 15 minutes (the vegetables should still be crunchy). Serve with plain yogurt and parsley on top.

Fruit Dip Dressing

Plain yogurt
lemon juice
honey
cinnamon
Mix to taste. Serve with apple wedges, grapes, banana chunks or strawberries.

RICE, MEXICAN STYLE

5 c. cooked brown rice
1 medium onion, diced
1/2 c. green pepper, diced
1/2 c. red pepper, diced
1/2 c. chopped green onions
1 c. mushrooms, sliced
2 cloves of garlic, pressed
1/4 c. canned green chilies
2 c. canned peeled tomatoes, chopped (and juice)
1/4 c. sliced black olives
2 t. chili powder
1 t. ground cumin
dash of hot sauce

Saute the onions, peppers, green onions and garlic lightly in one tablespoon of olive oil for a few minutes. Add mushrooms and saute a few minutes longer. Then add all remaining ingredients and stir. Cook five to ten minutes until it is heated thoroughly. Serve the vegetables over the rice.

SUMMER SALAD

1 c. fresh peas
4 carrots, thinly sliced
3 celery stalks, thinly sliced
6 radishes, sliced
1 green pepper, thinly sliced
6 green onions with stems
2 ears corn, cut off cob
4 c. cooked new potatoes, diced
1 c. lightly steamed green beans
Boston lettuce leaves
3 large tomatoes, cut in thin slices

Add all ingredients together, except the tomatoes. Chill in refrigerator. Toss all ingredients with herb vinaigrette dressing. Arrange mixture into salad bowl, lined with washed lettuce leaves. Garnish with sliced tomatoes and sunflower seeds if desired. Add vegetable seasoning or kelp to taste.

❖

THERMOS COOKING

Thermos cooking is an excellent way to supply nutrients to the body that are lacking in the typical American diet. Cooking in a thermos is a long slow gentle way to use grains without destroying the B-complex vitamins and enzymes, as well as vitamins. High heat cooking is destructive to whole grains.

A wide-mouthed thermos is ideal. It makes the food easier to remove. You rinse the thermos first with boiling water and spoon in the rinsed grain. Then fill to the top with boiling water, close the lid tightly and leave to cook overnight. There will be plenty of water-space to take care of expansion. Use the extra juice to drink, it is full of enzymes and vitamins and will be healing for the digestive tract.

For grains use 1/2 cup to 1 and 1/2 cups of boiling water. This works well for a pint thermos. Wash the grain well and drain off water. Put the grain in the thermos and to scald the grain pour in boiling water and leave a few minutes to heat both the grain and the thermos. Drain again, and leave the grain in the thermos. Fill to the top with boiling water, close the thermos tightly and leave twelve hours (overnight) for most varieties of grains.

Mixed Grains: Mix the following grains: buckwheat, whole oats, hard wheat, rye and whole barley. Use 1/2 cup of this mixture with 1 1/2 cup of boiling water.

Whole Wheat: Use 1/2 cup wheat to 1 1/2 cups water. For a quart thermos use 1 cup of wheat to 3 cups of water. The results are excellent using the directions above.

Brown Rice: A nice treat for breakfast. In a pint thermos use 1/2 cup to 1 1/2 cups boiling water.

Buckwheat: Use 1/2 cup buckwheat groats to 1 1/2 cups water. Takes only two hours to cook in thermos, but can be left overnight.

Barley: Use 1/2 cup barley and use the method above. It will cook in twelve hours.

Millet: This cereal needs to be brought to the boiling point and simmered for five minutes before putting in the thermos or the hard hulls will not be broken. Millet is an alkaline cereal and is easily assimilated and digested. Cook it half and half with brown rice.

11

CHIROPRACTIC AND HYDROTHERAPY

WHAT IS CHIROPRACTIC?

The philosophy of chiropractic handed down since it was founded by Daniel David Palmer (in 1895) is that chiropractic is first a preventive form of health care and only secondarily a curative form. Palmer put together a synthesis of Hippocrates, Plato, Aristotle, Galen and Vesalius with a proposition which taught that (1) we should look to the spine for the cause of disease (a Hippocratic admonition) because (2) it contains and protects the spinal cord, through which vital forces flow and are mediated to all parts of the body through the spinal nerves. Therefore, chiropractic is designed to restore the normal function of the nerve system. One chiropractor put it this way: "All I do is normalize the body."

Every cell of your body receives nerve impulses either directly or indirectly from the spine. Each one of these large nerve cables leaving the spine carries some 300,000 tiny nerves. The therapy of chiropractic is based upon the theory that disease is caused by interference with nerve functions. The goal of chiropractic, then, is concerned with freeing the interference of bodily processes caused by blocked or damaged nerve control which render the body less resistant to infection. This is true prevention for chiropractic attempts to enable the nervous system to perform its purposes of controlling and coordinating every cell, organ and structure in the body and to adapt the organism to its environment. The breakdown of the immunological systems and possible cancer can be avoided in the main, if the body is free to do what it was created to do.

Chiropractic calls these interferences subluxations (vertebral misalignment), and these are caused by birth, auto accidents, home accidents, practical jokes and horseplay, trauma and fear, falls, toxins from food additives, tobacco, alcohol, exhaust fumes and drugs. The subluxation is considered the main cause of disease, while the point at which the disease becomes apparent is the symptom.

TRAINING OF CHIROPRACTORS

Much of the criticism against chiropractic stems from ignorance of chiropractic training. Chiropractic students spend 4,485 hours studying many of the same things medical students (4,248 hours) study: anatomy, physiology, pathology, chemistry, bacteriology, diagnosis, neurology, x-ray, psychiatry, orthopedics (gynecology). Medical doctors also study pharmacology, immunology, and general surgery, but since chiropractors have a different philosophy of health, they receive training in adjusting, manipulation, and kinesiology instead. A student in chiropractic concentrates not on germs, but on improving the soil conditions of the body. He will see germs not as the prime cause of disease but as scavengers which exist to rid the body of morbid material, just as insects prey upon diseased plant life. In addition, he sees each individual patient as being biochemically unique. Yet within this uniqueness is a similarity anatomically and physiologically which enables the chiropractor to use his science.

As to those supporters of medical science who continue to call chiropractic an unscientific cult, the reader should remember that not only does the medical field espouse a different philosophy of medicine (treatment of symptoms rather than cause), it wants to have a monopoly on health care simply because it is so myopically sure that its way is the only way. Using medical bias it is certainly possible to prove that chiropractic is a false theory, or that educational standards are below that of MDs, or that it is dangerous. Each of these reasons has more holes than Swiss cheese, particularly the latter: any health care can be dangerous in the

❖

hands of he who practices not from compassion on the human condition, but simply from greed. Drug overdoses, complications from surgery, and malpractice suits are much more common among medical doctors than among any other kind of health practitioner.

TREATMENT

Although a chiropractor appears to be working primarily with the bones your spine and skeletal system, he knows this is merely the best approach to freeing the nerves so that they may perform the natural work for which they were naturally intended. This is why some people call chiropractors nerve specialists, rather than bone doctors. The bones and skeleton are merely the keys to open the doors to the nerves.

Many chiropractors practice nutrition counseling along with their chiropractic since it has been found that a well-fed person responds to any helpful therapy better than the poorly fed. Your chiropractor may supplement spinal adjustments and nutrition with electricity; water treatments; heat and cold; shoe, bed, seat or work position changes; acupressure; massage; kinesiology; vitamin therapy; traction; rehabilitative exercises and, above all, a re-education into the basics of health—which MD's normally don't provide.

WHAT IS HYDROTHERAPY?

Water is one of the best healers in existence. It is not irritating to use internally, it is good on the skin, and the only time you need to be careful is with extremes of temperatures on some people.

Water affects the entire body—muscles, nerves and liver. It can enhance the conversion of lactic acid from fatigued muscles back into useful energy. It also makes skin sensations more alive. Therapy with water can be used generally in two ways: hot or warm water and cold or cool water.

Hot or warm water dilates or expands the blood vessels that increase the speed of the blood's flow. Local application increases capillary pressure, the flow of fluid into the lymph spaces, perspiration, and also relieves pain. A warm bath relieves muscle fatigue and promotes sleep and rest.

❖

Cool or cold water when accompanied by rubbing and massage, stimulates the blood and the nerves. It begins a vascular gymnastics with the blood vessels pumping vigorously, alternating between dilation and contraction. For this reason never use cold water with exhaustion—your body won't be able to handle it. Cold delivers extra oxygen to the skin. Following a warm bath, a cold shower gives the body new energy, making the brain more alert and the extremities warmer. You will find that you will be able to accomplish more work.

There are many helpful techniques for the water to heal, soothe, stimulate or relax. The following are guidelines to incorporating these techniques.

FOMENTATIONS (WARM)
• relieve congestion of chest colds
• ease pain of arthritis
• stimulate (alternate with cola)
• sedate (use on spine)

HOT FOOT BATH (100-115 DEGREES)
• increase circulation
• heighten nerve and muscle tone, skin sensitivity
• increase antibody production

SITZBATH
• *Cold* (55-75 degrees)hemorrhoids, prostate, perinium and rectum surgery
• *Hot* (105-110 degrees) treat pelvic pain during menstrual cycle, inflammatory conditions. Use cold compresses to the head and neck simultaneously.

CONTRAST BATHS (HOT THEN COLD)
• poor circulation
• arthritis

ICE PACKS
• Eye injury, swelling, anesthetics

TUB BATHS
- Neutral (94-98 degrees)—sedative (cover the patient to the neck with a pillow under the neck)

There are other means to using water externally: epsom salts bath, sauna or steam bath, hot baths, warm baths, local wet pack, cool baths, cold baths, wet pack treatment, cold sheet treatment (Dr. Henry Lindlahr) and sulphur or pine baths. However you choose to use water as a method for improving health, Father Kneipp, the pioneer of hydrotherapy, would be proud of you for using such a simple, common technique for what ails you. And don't forget water's internal uses: douches, enemas, colonics, eye baths and mouth treatment.

SKIN BRUSHING

Regular bathing and washing will not remove the layers of dead skin. It takes a gentle and light abrasion on the skin when it is dry to rid the body of the dead unwanted skin. The dead layers need to be peeled away so the skin will be able to breath and live properly. This is what is referred to as dry skin brushing. Acne, pimples, excessive dryness or oiliness can all be greatly helped by this activity. It increases rapid cell production beneath the surface of the skin. It is considered the same body stimulation as compared to twenty minutes jogging or fast walking. Rubbing the skin with a turkish towel will make sure the lymphatic system and bloodstream are exercised. Use a skin brush made from natural bristles, with a long but detachable handle so that you can reach your back. It is a wonderful feeling, and so stimulating to brush just before you shower. It leaves a tingling and refreshing feeling.

Skin brushing is an effective way for cleansing the lymphatic system through physically stimulation. It also stimulates the bloodstream and is excellent for poor circulation and is a must on a colon cleansing program. It helps to dislodge mucus in the area that is needed. Start by brushing the soles of the feet and work up each leg, up the bottom and up to the middle of the back, (avoid the genitals). Work towards the heart and bring all toxins toward the colon. Then start at the fingertips and brush up the arms, across the shoulders, down the chest and the top of the back, again avoiding sensitive parts like the nipples. Don't forget

✛

the arm pits, this is where glandular inflammation collect in the lymph. Then brush down towards the colon. On the area below the navel, brush in movements starting on the right hand side, going up, across and down, following the shape of the colon. Women should brush the breasts, it cleans and protects against lumps. The face should always be cleaned with a wash cloth or a natural soft brush.

Another type of skin brushing or a brisk scrub is with stone ground corn meal while the skin is wet, followed by a tepid or cold rinse. This thoroughly cleanses the skin while stimulating circulation. The natural oil in the corn meal prevents irritation and leaves the skin baby soft.

12

ACUTE AND CHRONIC AILMENTS

Our present system recognizes disease only when it has reached crisis proportions. This is tantamount to saying that a fire is fire when it has burst through the roof, when in actuality, it was a fire when the cigarette butt began to smolder in the rug.

Carlton Fredericks

Disease is a warning. It is a friend, not a foe, of mankind. It manifests itself in its various forms, from a slight cold to the more severe inflammations, for the sole purpose of riding the body of accumulated poisons.

Dr. Wager, *The Law of Disease*

Nature provides a built-in cleansing mechanism, which is sometimes misinterpreted as a negative symptom because it manifests itself in the form of an acute disease. Dr. Henry Lindlahr, a medical doctor in the early 1900s, was considered an expert on this subject. His works constantly ring of logic and truth. His fundamental laws of cure, which form the basic principles of the science of natural healing, show that acute disease itself is a cure. It represents Nature's efforts to purify and regenerate the system.

What is an acute disease? Acute diseases have a rapid onset and run a short course and a short period of distress and discomfort, as compared to chronic disease. Chronic disease has a slow onset and lasts for a long period of time.

Common Acute Diseases

The following are common acute diseases: appendicitis, asthma, bladder infections, boils, Bright's disease, bronchitis, chicken pox, colds, congestion of the kidneys, coughs, croup, cystitis, diarrhea, diphtheria, dysentery, ear infections, endocarditis, enteritis, eye infections, gastritis, German measles, glaucoma, gout, gonorrhea, hayfever, hemorrhages, hives, hydrophobia, influenza, jaundice, laryngitis, lung problems, mumps, nephritis, phlebitis, pleurisy, pneumonia, scarlet fever, syphilis, smallpox, tetanus, tonsillitis, toothache, typhoid fever, tuberculosis, whooping cough, and yellow fever.

Colds, flu and fevers are a natural eliminative process—a safety valve which the body opens of its own accord to give it a chance to eradicate toxins. A short fast will help hasten the stage of acute disease. Use lemon, lime, grapefruit and orange juices diluted with pure water; also, you may use herbal teas. No sweet juices such as grape or apple should be used during an acute disease, as they cause fermentation in the intestinal tract. Acute disease is a healing and cleansing of the body, so the body is really trying to eliminate from the cells and organs the accumulated toxins and poisons. It brings them to the stomach to be eliminated. Cleansing is stopped when you eat food because the body has to use its energy to digest it. People usually feel better when this natural cleanse is stopped because their "aches" and "pains" go away for a while. Eating, however, will stop this vital process and will drive the mucus and toxins deeper into the body, where it will take a greater cleanse next time to get rid of them. Eating will deplete the body of energy to heal.

Why do people catch colds after they are chilled? Dr. Lindlahr explains: "Taking cold may be caused by chilling the surface of the body or part of the body. In the chilled portions of the skin the pores close; the blood recedes into the interior, and as a result, the elimination of poisonous gases and exudates is locally suppressed. This catching cold through being exposed to a cold draft, through wet clothing, etc., is not necessarily followed by more serious consequences. If the system is not much encumbered with morbid matter and if the kidneys and intestines are in fairly good working order, these organs will assist the temporarily inactive skin to take care of the extra amount of waste and morbid materials and eliminate them without difficulty. The greater the vitality and the more normal the composition of the blood, the more effectively the system as a whole will react in such an emergency and throw off the morbid materials which were not eliminated through the skin."

Acute diseases are nature's therapy of cleansing and healing the system. The body will respond to this healing if certain rules are followed. Fasting from solid food will help nature do her job. Drinking lemon juice in pure water or herbal teas is one way to assist nature. Using herbs is an excellent way to assist nature, depending upon the symptoms the acute disease manifests. An herbal lower bowel cleanser helps to clean and restore bowel function by eliminating toxins. When we allow nature to do its job, acute diseases will help prevent chronic diseases in the future.

The following excerpt is from a book by Henry Lindlahr, M.D., *Philosophy of Natural Therapeutics,* published in 1918:

> Smallpox, like every other infectious disease, is a filth disease; its microzyma grow in morbid soil only and that the smallpox eruptions are a sign of rapid elimination of hereditary and acquired disease taints.
>
> A good dose of smallpox may rid the system of more scrofulous, tuberculous and syphilitic poisons than could otherwise be gotten rid of in a lifetime. Therefore smallpox is certainly to be preferred to vaccination. The one means the elimination of chronic disease, the other making of it.
>
> "Cheap talk!" someone says. Not so, my friend! This is not mere talk. I was put to the test in the case of my own family and therefore speak from personal experience. My oldest boy was born at a time when both parents were heavily encumbered with hereditary and acquired disease conditions. At birth he weighed only two and a half pounds and his chance for life seemed very slight. The eyes were of a blackish blue, especially the outer portion of the iris, and this gradually condensed into a heavy scurf rim owing to the fact that nature's cleansing efforts in the form of skin eruptions were promptly suppressed with talcum powder and other home remedies.
>
> For the first five or six years of his life our boy was a weak, sickly child, having one after another all of the common infantile ailments. However, we soon learned to treat these natural methods and he was not vaccinated.
>
> One day suspicious looking eruptions appeared, which soon spread all over his body. I called in two allopathic physicians to verify my own diagnosis of smallpox, which they did unqualifiedly.
>
> We applied the natural treatment, which consisted of strict fasting, colon flushing and cold water applications. The child was kept day and

night in wet packs—strips of linen wrung out of water of natural temperature and covered with flannel bandages which were changed whenever they became hot and dry. The face also was kept covered with cooling compresses. In addition to this treatment I gave the indicated high potency homeopathic remedies. There was hardly a spot on the boy's body that was not covered with sores. However, constant renewal of the cold packs kept the temperature below the danger point and greatly alleviated the insufferable itching peculiar to the disease.

My wife, her sister and myself by turns slept in the same room with the child without the least fear of infection, and although we had not been vaccinated since childhood we remained unaffected by the contagious disease.

The wet packs, of course, greatly furthered the processes of elimination, and the disease practically ran its course in ten days. From that time on the sores healed rapidly and nothing remained to indicate the "ravages" of the disease but a telltale mark over the left eyebrow and a few similar scars on the boy's body. These also have now entirely disappeared.

Under this natural treatment of the disease convalescence was rapid and complete, and soon after the eyes became much clearer and much lighter in color. Since his recovery from the smallpox this boy has never had a sick day. He is now in his twenty-first year and well developed physically and mentally.

As far as I could learn, there was not another case of smallpox in Chicago and vicinity at the time of the boy's illness. If the infection theory be true, from whom did he catch the disease and why did not one of the many persons living in the same house become infected? My answer is: "This acute eliminative process was Nature's way of purifying the little body of inherited scrofulous and other disease taints."

Dr. Lindlahr taught and proved in his medical practice that all acute diseases are the same in nature and purpose and that they run the same course through five stages of inflammation. These stages are incubation, aggravation, destruction, abatement and reconstruction. All five stages are necessary for complete cleansing and subsequent healing of the body. Every disease, whether it is acute or chronic, has to go through five stages of inflammation. This is a natural law.

Some people think that they are healthy because they never get "sick." Yet they have improper diets and allow stress to bind them up. These people need to initiate a cleanse by going on the same program as those who come down with the acute diseases. Persons who eat devitalized foods and who go year after year without a "housecleaning" may find themselves someday with a full blown chronic disease and wonder where it came from.

STAGES I AND II:
INCUBATION AND AGGRAVATION

These stages occur when the body is trying to eliminate toxic material through an acute disease. The energy and nutrients of the body are depleted from stress, personal problems and life, and bad eating habits. The body is unable to eliminate toxins, poisons, drugs, etc., and they accumulate in the tissues, causing an obstruction at some point. This period may last from a few hours to several days, weeks, months, or even years. During this stage, waste matter, poisons, pollution, germs, parasites and other uninvited guests congregate in certain parts and organs of the body. When they have accumulated to such an extent as to interfere with the normal functions of life or to endanger the health and life of the body, the life forces begin to react to the obstruction or threatening danger by creating the inflammatory process. The body is unable to resist and does not have the energy or power to overcome the natural attraction to germs. Vitality reserve is low, and has been all used up. If the toxins and mucus are not eliminated, they are thrown further into the organs of the body and will buildup in the joints, the organs, the lymphatic system and around the heart and veins and start to solidify for chronic conditions of the body. The tonsils and appendix protect the body and help in the eliminating process in acute diseases. If they have been surgically removed, then the body has to work harder to get rid of waste matter and toxins, through the lymphatics and liver. If cleansing is suppressed at this stage (through eating or taking drugs), then mucus, toxins and pus will harden in the body for chronic conditions of the organs.

STAGE III:
DESTRUCTION

This stage is where the battle between the immune system and the toxins of disease gradually progresses, accompanied by a corresponding increase of fever and inflamed tissues where they can incubate into

❖

chronic conditions. Also, there is a lot of pus and mucus in the body, when tissues are being broken down. The organs at this stage are holding pus, mucus, and toxins and retaining them in the organs. When the body is suppressed by drugs and eating, the toxins stay in the organs and cause pneumonia, tuberculosis, infantile paralysis, spinal meningitis, asthma, emphysema, bronchitis and many other diseases. Using natural methods will assist nature in eliminating toxins without causing serious damage.

STAGE IV:
ABATEMENT STAGE

This stage is where the body begins to eliminate excess waste. The body is now strong enough to win the battle. Appropriate treatment will build up the blood, increase the vitality and promote natural elimination. Then the poisons and germs of disease will be overcome and eliminated. The glands in the system are absorbing all the excess waste as in the lymphatic glands and the intestinal glands. The fever reduces, and the symptoms decrease. As they are being absorbed and with the right treatment, the body will expel the toxins. If the cleansing is suppressed at this stage, the glands will become congested. This will result in lymphatic congestion, glandular secretions, tumors, cysts, moles and skin diseases. This stage sets the environment for all diseases.

STAGE V:
RECONSTRUCTION

When the period of absorption has run its course and the affected areas have been cleared of the morbid accumulations and obstructions, then during the fifth stage of inflammation, the work of rebuilding begins. The struggle has been more or less destructive to the cells, tissues, blood vessels and organs of the areas involved. They must now be reconstructed, and this last stage of inflammatory process is, therefore, in a way the most important.

This is the process of regeneration of the injured parts of the body. If the process of reconstruction is interfered with or interrupted before it is completed, the microzyma will continue to create germs of putrefaction and the affected parts and organs will not have a chance to become entirely clean, well or strong. The body will remain in an abnormal, diseased condition and its functional activity will be seriously handicapped.

The body is still weak during Stage V and has a lot of poisons. This is the building stage, and if a disease is suppressed at this time, the absorption glands remain full. They swell up, then they shrink and cannot produce the hormones properly. Now we have low hormone output, low lymphatic absorption, and the intestinal tract is still coated. We experience indigestion, anemia and deficiencies in the body, and an imbalance is created. We cannot absorb our nutrients properly. We have suppressed an acute disease at the stage where we should be restoring the cells with the proper environment for chronic disease, and now we are told they are incurable diseases. The diseases we are treating now are AIDS, leukemia, all kinds of cancer, candida, diabetes, herpes, Epstein-Barr, etc.

When treating acute diseases with natural methods such as cleaning the bowels, fasting (stop eating), citrus juices and herbal teas, water therapy, fresh air, rest and some physical manipulation—it will always be best if the five stages are allowed to run their natural course.

Dr. Lindlahr maintained that natural remedies can be applied from the first sign of an acute disease, at the slightest manifestation of inflammatory and fever symptoms. One of the principles that he stressed is that prevention is better than the cure. Orthodox medical science has learned that this is true as far as surroundings are concerned, but has not yet applied this principal to internal conditions. The theory espoused by modern medical science is to "kill the germ and cure the disease." With the drugs they prescribe they have developed drug therapies that suppress the acute disease. This complicates the condition and/or throws it deeper into the organs to cause a chronic disease later.

The first temporary violent effect of poisonous drugs, in active doses, is usually due to nature's effort to overcome and eliminate these substances. Continued use of drugs often results in complete exhaustion and paralysis of mental and physical powers. Each drug breeds new disease symptoms, which are in their turn, "cured" by other poisons until the body is too weak to throw off the toxins and drugs.

If we use drugs or food, they will suppress the flu or cold, and that which should have been eliminated will be retained within the body. As

❖

long as we continue to suppress the natural process of elimination, the toxic material will begin to settle in the organs of the body to eventually create what we call chronic disease, such as arthritis, diabetes, chronic asthma, etc.

We must emphasize that you can eat a highly nutritious diet and still create a toxic condition in your body. How is that? Well, if you allow negative emotions to breed inside and take root, this will affect the function of your body. The stress will upset your organs and glands and will turn the food you ingest into toxic substances. Hate, especially, is such a strong emotion that it will wreak havoc and turmoil inside of you by producing toxic acids. It will jeopardize your immune system. You can see what stress can do to you if you are in a weakened condition. If junk food is consumed, with no regard to healthful eating habits or supplements, then the body cannot become fortified to handle stress. We must learn to cultivate a positive attitude, as well as discipline ourselves to eat foods with high-nutrient density. Proper bowel management, cleansing and a positive mental attitude can contribute to a longer, healthier life.

A-Z AILMENT LISTING

❖ ABSCESS

Abscesses include boils, carbuncles (a large boil with multiple heads), felon or whitlow. A boil on the edge of the eye is called a sty. An abscess is a localized, inflamed area due to infection. It has an accumulation of white, yellow or green pus. It is nature's way of isolating, cleaning and eliminating infections. They are usually found just beneath the skin, although they can be found anywhere, such as in the brain, lungs, gums, teeth, ears, tonsils, sinuses, breasts, kidneys or in any part of the body. Boils start as a raised patch of skin, then turn red or purple, and become swollen and painful. An imbalance in the body can cause boils as is impure blood and poor fat metabolism is one cause. Frequent recurring boils may indicate problems such as diabetes.

❖

The skin is the body's largest elimination organ, constantly eliminating acids, gases, vapors and toxins. When the skin becomes congested it is usually caused from toxins in the urinary tract. Skin problems and urinary tract infections go hand in hand. People who have skin problems will usually have kidney and bladder problems. The filtering system of the kidneys becomes clogged with built-up mucus, and needs to be dissolved for better elimination.

Dr. Robert S. Mendelsohn said that the most common cause of rectal abscess in babies is severe constipation. This goes along with the skin trying to eliminate when the kidneys and colon are congested. Babies can be born with poor colon function.

Natural Therapy: Cleansing the blood using natural, herbal antibiotics. A lower bowel cleanser will speed up the removal of toxins, juice fasts, eating a lot of fresh salads; stay with the alkaline foods.

External: Slippery elm, black walnut and fenugreek poultice in a powdered form, moistened with aloe vera juice or pure water. (Apply externally to help dissolve abscesses and boils). Lemon juice applied externally and taken internally with pure water. A poultice made with charcoal and water will help draw out the poisons. Use a clean piece of cotton.

Foods to Heal: Vegetables and fruits, raw and lightly steamed are excellent as are fresh vegetable juices (carrot, celery) and vegetable green drinks. Citrus fruits and juices are cleansing, (limes, lemons, oranges and grapefruit). Carrots, apricots, parsley, sprouts, yellow fruits and vegetables, cherries, green peppers, broccoli, red cabbage, berries, papaya, asparagus, leaf lettuce, pineapple, sweet potatoes, winter squash, oats, millet, brown rice, sesame seeds, blackstrap molasses, almonds, pumpkin seeds, barley, potatoes, yams are good for healing.

Vitamins and Minerals: Vitamin A (large amounts for a week), B-complex vitamins speed healing, vitamin C with bioflavonoids speeds healing, and vitamin E can be used to avoid external scarring. Multimineral supplements, especially with extra calcium and magnesium balance, manganese, silicon, selenium and zinc (50 to 100 mg per day) are very healing.

Herbal Combination: For internal abscess, use blood purifier, antibiotic

❖

and lower-bowel formulas. For external abscess, use black herbal ointment, or a goldenseal ointment.

Single Herbs: Aloe vera (heals scar tissue, boils leave scars), burdock (antibiotic and blood cleanser), black walnut, capsicum, chaparral, echinacea (heals and cleans blood), garlic (natural antibiotic), ginger, goldenseal, (antiseptic, and antibiotic), horsetail, kelp, marshmallow (use internally and as a poultice), myrrh, pau d'arco, parsley, plantain (soothes inflammation and heals scar tissues), red clover (blood purifier), slippery elm (contains demulcent properties, healing), yarrow, yellow dock.

Supplements: Acidophilus, bee pollen, blue-green algae (increases oxygen utilization and protects against viral infections), liquid chlorophyll, flaxseed poultice and clay packs, chinese essential formula, tea tree oil, and essential fatty acids such as salmon oil and evening primrose oil (protect the immune system).

Avoid: Sugar, and all sugar products; white flour and pastry; meat and cheese; fried foods; and antibiotics (weaken the immune system). Avoid a high-fat diet, chocolate, pastries, candy, cookies, ice cream and all soft drinks.

❖ ADDICTION

Addiction may be mental or emotional. We may suspect addictions when there are repeated foods or substances we feel our body has to have at all times. Sugar is the underlying basis for most addictions. It gives us false energy. Mental work requires a lot of energy. We can add more fresh or dried fruits for more mental work. Industry puts sugar in almost all food. The following can be addictive: alcohol, coffee, tea, drugs, sugar, tobacco, chocolate, illegal drugs, over-the-counter drugs, caffeine drinks, and prescribed drugs.

Addictions are damaging to the brain, nervous system, digestion, liver and pancreas. Alcohol and drugs destroy brain cells and weaken the hypothalamus (appetite control), creating a craving or addiction. The immune system is affected and it leaves the body open to all kinds of disease.

Addictions deplete the essential vitamins and minerals, while giving a false sense of energy. Excessive liquids eliminate minerals from the

❖

body as well as the B-complex vitamins. Junk food increases the body's dependency on addictions but does not satisfy the body's need for nutrients. Hypoglycemia is very often linked with addictions.

Natural Therapy: Cleanse the blood and strengthen the liver, digestion, and the nerves. Do this through juice fasts and green drinks, using carrots, celery, parsley and fresh apple juice. Skin brushing with hot and cold showers will cause sweating to help clean out the toxins. Steamed vegetables provide minerals to the body. Use pure water, vegetable broths and a lot of fruit and vegetable salads.

Foods to Heal: Yellow fruits and vegetables, green leafy vegetables, vegetable juices, and grains (thermos cooking to retain the B-complex vitamins and enzymes). Wheat grass juice is healing. Those who have been heavy meat eaters can substitute meat with grains. Buckwheat, millet, brown rice, whole oats, wheat, and barley. Beans are nourishing. Nuts, seeds and sprouts of all kinds will help supply the body natural nutrients. Roasted grain drinks help with coffee addictions. A balanced diet will satisfy the body's need and help control addictions.

Vitamins and Minerals: Vitamin A strengthens the immune system and protects the lungs), B-complex calms the nerves, vitamin C is a cleanser and healer, calcium calms the nerves, selenium, and zinc, which is depleted in addictions. Multimineral supplements will strengthen the whole body.

Herbal Combinations: Digestion, glands, heart, liver and nerves.

Single Herbs: Alfalfa, black cohosh, black walnut, burdock (purifies the blood), capsicum, chaparral, dandelion (protects and nourishes the liver), echinacea (cleans the lymphatics and blood), garlic, gentian (cleans and heals the digestive system), ginger, ginkgo (strengthens the whole body), goldenseal (healing and purifying), gotu kola (strengthens the brain), hawthorn (improves heart function), ho-shou-wu (improves energy output), hops (builds the nerves), kelp, licorice, lobelia, milk thistle, pau d'arco, passionflower, red clover (cleans the blood and liver), saffron (helps in digestion of fats), skullcap, valerian and wood betony.

Supplements: Evening primrose oil, salmon oil, rice bran syrup, liquid chlorophyll, herbal teas (rich in minerals), teas that contain nervine

❖

herbs (chamomile, hops, skullcap, catnip), and grain drinks (substitute for coffee).

Avoid: Sugar (increases addictions), try to eliminate meat if possible, especially beef (accumulates hormones, antibiotics, and uric acid in the body). Avoid all food and drugs that may cause a dependency, including nicotine, alcohol, caffeine, and marijuana. Caffeine and sugar together are addictive and they give a false sense of energy.

❖ AGING

Aging is a natural process that gradually develops from the time you are born. It is a state that is usually arrived at slowly, but life stresses can determine an early aging process. Premature aging can develop with constant sickness, exhaustion and stresses of life.

Although we cannot avoid aging we can control the diseases that accompany old age. Chronological age is determined by years of existence. Physical or biological age is determined by functional activity and is a true indicator of true age and quality of life.

The thymus gland shrinks under stress and it is the master gland of the immune system. The nutrients that nourish the thymus are essential to longevity and health. Lifestyle change in the areas of diet and exercise can add years to your life as well as increase happiness through good health. It doesn't matter how long you live as long as you are happy and healthy.

Use correct food combining for proper nutrition. Eat less food, but choose it wisely. A single nutrient deficiency can result in a faulty immune system and determine our response to disease. The happiest and most active elderly Americans are the ones that eat healthy and have more mental and physical energy.

Natural Therapy: Keep the blood clean, the bowels open and the glands fed. Exercise physically as well as mentally. A positive attitude protects the immune system. Increased supplements are needed along with digestive enzymes and hydrochloric acid to assure assimilation of supplements and food.

Foods to Heal: High-quality protein and amino acids (soy milk drinks), millet and buckwheat, raw vegetables, fruits, grains, seeds, nuts and sprouts. Eat a lot of broccoli, cabbage, cauliflower, and fiber foods (psyllium). Cut down on fats and sugar products.

Vitamins and Minerals: Vitamins A, C, and E, along with the trace mineral selenium, are all natural antioxidants. They destroy free radicals and protect against toxins, viruses, bacteria, smog and radiation. Vitamin D increases absorption of minerals in the bones and calcium from the stomach. Vitamin B-complex is important, especially B_6, pantothenic acid folic acid and B_{12}. Deficiencies are seen in the elderly. Vitamin C is essential for the production of interferon that destroys viruses and it protects cells and heals wounds. Vitamin E increases resistance to disease. Selenium protects against cancer and improves antibody production. Zinc builds the immune system and is healing for wounds. All vitamins and minerals work together. Calcium can be obtained from an herbal calcium formula and minerals from herbs such as alfalfa, kelp and dulse.

Herbal Combinations: Bone, chelation formula (cleans the veins), digestion, endurance, glands and immune combinations.

Single Herbs: Alfalfa, cayenne, damiana, dong quai (strengthens all female organs), eyebright (cleans and protects the eyes), false unicorn, garlic (protects the veins and immune system), gentian, ginkgo (strengthens blood vessels, increases blood flow to brain), ginseng (strengthens whole body, prevents senility), gotu kola (improves memory and brain function), hawthorn (builds heart muscles and dilates blood vessels), hops, horsetail, (calcium), ho-shou-wu (improves health, stamina), kelp (chelates metals), lady's slipper, licorice (increases energy), lobelia, oatstraw, papaya, pau d'arco, red clover, sarsaparilla, suma (immune system booster), yellow dock (rich in plant iron), yucca (cleans deep in the cells).

Supplements: Bee pollen and spirulina (RNA-DNA), evening primrose oil, fish oil lipids, salmon oil, lecithin (choline and inositol), royal jelly (dilates and strengthens blood vessels, rebuilds tissue, and feeds the glands), whey powder (help joints remain limber and prevents calcium deposits), blue-green algae (provides oxygen to the cells and builds the immune system).

Avoid: Processed foods, coffee, tea, cocoa, caffeine drinks. Alcohol dilates the blood vessels and causes weak veins. Excessive consump-

❖

tion of soft drinks can deplete calcium, because of its high content of phosphorus. Increases bone problems such as osteoporosis. Chlorinated water speeds the aging process. Avoid salt, fats and sugar. Also avoid tobacco, red meat, alcohol, coffee, tea and caffeine drinks.

❖ AIDS (ACQUIRED IMMUNE DEFICIENCY SYNDROME)

With this disease, the immune system is completely broken down by a virus and is complicated by other disorders which accompany it. This is indeed a modern day plague.

Dr. Eva Snead, M.D., extensively researched AIDS and discovered that some viral vaccines are made in the kidney of the African green monkey. She explains that the African green monkey contains hundreds of viruses and the monkey cells are loaded with the AIDS virus. She discovered that the AIDS virus was developed in a laboratory from the kidney of the African green monkey, and that the World Health Organization (WHO) had "triggered" the AIDS epidemic in Africa through the WHO smallpox immunization program. The WHO vaccinated 37 million in Zaire, 19 million in Zambia, 15 million in Tanzania, 12 million in Uganda and 8 million in Malawi. It is estimated that one third of the African population could have the disease within the next six years.

The majority of people in the world get immunized—about four billion total. Why is Africa harboring AIDS? Could there be a connection between vaccinations and AIDS? In Dr. Douglass' book, *AIDS: The End Of Civilization,* he calls AIDS "the greatest biological disaster in the history of mankind." I am inclined to believe him. We are seeing too many people with AIDS, and other immune related diseases. Snead says that everyone who has been vaccinated has the AIDS virus in them as well as forty other viruses, including the Epstein Barr virus.

Foods to Heal: The best type of diet is 80 percent raw food, especially foods high in vitamins A and C such as fish liver oils, yellow vegetables and fruits, citrus fruits, strawberries, kale, alfalfa sprouts, papaya, broccoli, parsley and wheat grass. Onions, garlic, cabbage, turnips, winter squash are also highly nutritious. Use kelp, paprika and herbs for seasoning, along with fresh lemon juice and cold-pressed oils. Use millet or rice cakes instead of bread. Use millet, brown rice, buckwheat and wild rice dishes. Sprouts will provide live enzymes to help supply nutrients.

Vitamins and Minerals: Use multivitamins with extra vitamins A, B-complex, C with bioflavonoids, D, and E (builds up the immune system). Multiminerals with extra calcium are desirable because an herbal calcium will supply silicon for calcium assimilation. Also include selenium and zinc.

Herbal Combinations: Blood purifier, digestion, infection, immune, liver, lower bowels and nerve formulas. A garlic anti-plague formula will protect and build the immune system.

Single Herbs: Black walnut (expels worms and balances minerals), burdock (cleans the blood), cayenne, chaparral (cleans deep into the cells), echinacea (cleans the lymphatics for pure blood), garlic (a natural antibiotic), goldenseal (cleans the digestive system for better assimilation), kelp, marshmallow, milk thistle (heals and restores liver function), pau d'arco (cleans blood and protects the liver), red clover (blood purifier), sarsaparilla, skullcap, suma (strengthens the whole body) and wormwood.

Supplements: Acidophilus, algin, bee pollen, caprylic acid, evening primrose oil, lecithin, spirulina, wheat grass juice, green drinks and chlorophyll. Digestive enzymes and hydrochloric acid tablets to help in digestion and assimilation.

Avoid: Processed foods, salt, processed meats (bacon, hot dogs, etc.), white sugar, white flour and excessive dairy products (eggs, cheese, pasteurized milk). Avoid all pickled products such as salad dressings, green olives, and relishes. All dry roasted nuts, potato chips, pretzels, crackers, soda pop, bacon, salt pork, lunch meats and cheeses of all kinds should also be avoided. Stay away from leftover food where molds and yeast grow and thrive.

✤ ALLERGIES

Digestion problems and a faulty immune system can precipitate allergic reactions in the body. The body is sensitive and reacts to certain irritants, which otherwise would not affect it. Allergic symptoms can range from the common hay fever type (sneezing, red eyes) to fatigue, irritability and myriads of other symptoms.

An easy way to determine if you have a food allergy is to relax, take the pulse of your wrist for sixty seconds and ecord the number of beats. Then eat the food you think you may be allergic to. After fifteen or twenty minutes, take your pulse again. If it increases more than ten beats per minute, you can suspect an allergy. Refrain from eating that food for one month, then eat it and test again. An average pulse reading is 52-70.

Causes of allergies are poor diet, with digestion and assimilation problems, with toxins being absorbed into the blood and lymphatic system, causing excess mucus. The excess mucus can be secreted in different areas of the body such as the nasal passages, bronchials, lungs, ears, eyes, or in the reproductive organs causing whitish or clear discharge.

Undigested proteins act as irritants in the body. The cells treat them as foreign invaders, thus inviting an allergic attack. An efficient digestive system is necessary to prevent accumulations of these substances in the bloodstream. Mucous membranes line many areas of the body—the nose, throat, most organs and glands and the gastrointestinal tract. Healthy mucous membranes will not allow the undigested proteins to enter the bloodstream.

The colon plays a vital function in preventing allergies. Its role is to eliminate waste material. However, due to faulty eating habits, eating junk food, or the wrong combination of foods, too much meat and an unbalanced diet, the colon becomes congested or constipated. It will then harbor all manner of toxins, which will poison the body when released into the blood stream. This state of autointoxication lowers immune capability of the body and sets the stage or condition for allergies to occur.

Natural Therapy: Blood purification and a cleansing diet is the best sort of therapy. Use food enzymes and hydrochloric acid to ensure complete digestion of food. The bowels must be kept clean. Do juice fasts using carrot, celery and raw apple juice. Liver cleanses may be necessary for when the liver is clogged with fats and accumulated toxins. It cannot produce histaminase, which protects the body from allergies. When the digestive system is functioning properly and the colon is working every day, allergies will gradually disappear.

Foods to Heal: Sprouts, almonds, beans, raw nuts, peas, lemons, sesame seeds, green leafy vegetables, root vegetables, buckwheat, yellow fruits and vegetables. berries, carrots, apricots, parsley, celery, cabbage, watercress, apples, grapes, onions, artichokes, and garlic. Magnesium foods that prevent allergies are almonds, whole grains, cashews, sesame seed, lima, white, and red beans, millet, bananas, wild rice, brown rice. Sodium is found in zucchini, celery, carrots, beets and seaweeds.

Vitamins and Minerals: Take multivitamins with extra A, B-complex (pantothenic acid, B_6, B_{12}) and vitamin C with bioflavonoids (helps in assimilation of iron). Take multiminerals with extra calcium and magnesium (prevents allergies), manganese, potassium, zinc. Iodine (found in kelp) is necessary to produce thyroid hormone and to protect metabolism. Sodium that is found naturally in herbs and food prevents water getting into the cells, which results in stuffy nose, watery eyes and swollen tissues. Pantothenic acid, vitamin C and vitamin E have all been shown to reduce the production of histamines under stress.

Herbal Combinations: Allergy, bone, digestion, lungs, lower bowel formulas. Herbal formulas will help clean and strengthen the mucous membranes.

Single Herbs: Alfalfa (acid/alkaline balance), burdock (with dandelion strengthens the liver), chaparral (cleans deep in the cells), chickweed, comfrey, dandelion, echinacea, eyebright, fenugreek (cleans the stomach of mucus), gentian (tonic for the intestinal tract), goldenseal (antibiotic, congestion), gotu kola (feeds the brain), hops (sedative, headaches), ho-shou-wu, Irish moss, lobelia, ma huang (natural antihistamine), myrrh, parsley, psyllium, red raspberry, skullcap, slippery elm, wood betony, wormwood, yellow dock.

Supplements: Amino acids (histidine, isoleucine, tryptophan, tyrosine), bee pollen, acidophilus (milk-free), bentonite, fish oil lipids, salmon oil, evening primrose oil (essential fatty acids are needed to produce adrenal hormones and to synthesize pantothenic acid in the intestines), rice bran syrup, royal jelly, glucomannan. Digestive enzymes to aid in digestion to prevent toxins from accumulating in the blood.

❖

Avoid: Any foods that provoke allergic symptoms (introduce back into diet one at a time after one month of complete abstention from them). Common allergenic foods include wheat products, corn products, chocolate, dairy products, white potatoes, tomatoes and tobacco (night shade family). Avoid MSG, nitrates, artificial food colors or flavors, chemically grown or sprayed foods (also grains), processed oils or refined flour. Strong spices overstimulates the adrenals. Stay away from sugar, coffee and alcohol.

❖ ALZHEIMER'S DISEASE

Alzheimer's disease is characterized by progressive degeneration of the brain, memory and nervous system. Studies indicate that high aluminum concentrations in the brain tissue may be one causative factor. Another may be the diminished activity of the neurotransmitter acetylcholine. Neurotransmitters are chemicals located at the ends of brain nerve cells which make message transmission possible.

This is a devastating disease that affects the families of the victims. It brings heartache, discomfort, frustration and hopelessness to those involved. New light and beliefs are being shed on diseases affecting the nervous system and brain. Many of these disorders can be prevented, delayed or controlled with nutritional supplements. The brain suffers when nutrients are lacking, especially the essential minerals. The brain is very susceptible to nutritional deficiencies and also to environmental toxins. It is also sensitive to toxins created in an unhealthy colon. An unhealthy bloodstream can carry toxins to the brain and nervous system and cause brain cells to die.

Natural Therapy: Oral chelation, using vitamins, minerals, herbs, amino acids have been successful in cleaning the veins. Choline, found in lecithin, stimulates production of acetylcholine and improves Alzheimer's victims short term memory. Cleansing the liver and the bowels is beneficial. A low-fat diet and exercise are helpful.

Foods to Heal: A high-fiber diet is important. Fresh fruits and vegetables, green leafy vegetable salads, using different kinds of cabbage (red, green, chinese), broccoli, asparagus, carrots, cauliflower, sprouts, seeds, nuts, cold pressed oils, lemons, oranges, grapefruit. Millet,

❖

buckwheat, brown rice, a lot of lightly steamed vegetables, fish. Sulphur foods act as chelating agents: Watercress, brussels sprouts, horseradish, cabbage, turnip, cauliflower, raspberry, spinach, kelp, parsnip, leeks, garlic, onions, chives, swiss chard, okra. Distilled water has a chelating effect on the veins.

Vitamins and Minerals: Take B-complex vitamins with extra thiamine, B_6, niacin, B_{15}. Vitamin C, calcium and magnesium may help reduce levels of aluminum as well as prevent it from accumulating. Vitamin E helps transport oxygen to the brain cells and may also lower the possibile onset of Alzheimer's. Minerals are essential for a healthy nervous system and brain. Copper, manganese, magnesium, iodine, silver and zinc play a vital role in memory and brain function. These are elements that are in some way interdependent, and it's not possible to determine which one is the most important. Selenium, iodine and potassium are also important for continued brain function. Sulphur is found and needed mostly in the nervous system and brain. It purifies and activates the body. Phosphorus nourishes the brain and nerves.

Herbal Combinations: Liver, lower bowels, immune, nerves, potassium. Stress and anti-plague formulas containing garlic help protect the immune system, which is also part of the nervous system and the brain.

Single Herbs: Alfalfa, burdock, butcher's broom (improves circulation), capsicum (supplies nutrients to the brain), chaparral, echinacea, garlic (dissolves cholesterol and loosens it out of arteries), ginger, ginseng (increases brain efficiency and improves concentration), ginkgo (strengthen brain function), gotu kola (feeds the brain), ho-shou-wu, lady's slipper (feeds the nervous system), passionflower, prickly ash (increases circulation and cleans veins), psyllium (helps clean the colon of toxins), rosemary, red clover, skullcap, suma (increases brain function), valerian, wood betony.

Supplements: Coenzyme Q_{10} (carries oxygen to brain), germanium (oxygen), lecithin, RNA nutrients (sardines, spirulina, chlorella and bee pollen), free-form amino acids, salmon oil, blue-green algae.

Avoid: Avoid all aluminum products. Aluminum is found in most baking powders, cheese sauces, pickles, many salad dressings, table salt,

❖

white flour, fruit juices stored in aluminum cans, water from most municipal sources. It is found in some medicines. It is found in aspirin, antiperspirants, douches and feminine hygiene products, lipstick, antidiarrheal medications, and antacids. It is also found in many other products. Avoid all foods that lower the immune system: sugar, white flour products, alcohol, tobacco, caffeine, additives and preservatives. Avoid red meat because its by-product is uric acid, and it is very hard to digest. If you use meat, obtain organically grown meat without antibiotics and hormones. Avoid all processed food— the body needs essential nutrients for a healthy brain and nervous system.

❖ ANEMIA

Symptoms of anemia include fatigue, loss of appetite, irritability, general weakness, pale skin and fingernails and headaches. Lack of or poor assimilation of B$_{12}$ or iron can cause anemia. Healthy blood is the life-line to all the organs of the body. An unbalanced diet, poor digestion, and wrong food combining adds up to poor blood and anemia.

Anemia can also occur from recurrent infections or diseases involving the entire body. It also can happen with excessive losses of blood through such conditions as heavy menstruation or peptic ulcers.

Natural Therapy: Use blood purifiers. The blood transports nutrients, hormones, electrolytes, and waste material to and from every cell in the body; an imbalance or lack of nutrients leads to many problems and symptoms. Herbal therapies can benefit the glands, circulatory system and digestive tract.

Foods to Heal: Whole grains, blackberries, cherries, blackstrap molasses, dried apricots (rich in iron), peaches, raisins, prunes, sunflower seeds, sesame seeds, egg yolks, fish, sprouts, beets, millet, buckwheat, yams, sweet potatoes, squash, plums, potatoes (with skins), red cabbage. Enjoy all natural food, using a variety of fresh fruit, vegetables and sprouts. Fresh green salads will nourish and feed the blood.

Vitamins and Minerals: Iron, protein, copper, folic acid and vitamins B$_6$, B$_{12}$, and C are all essential for the formation of red blood cells. Vitamin E may be needed to help maintain the health of the red blood cells. Vitamins A, B-complex (extra B$_6$, B$_{12}$, PABA and pantothenic acid), C (with bioflavonoids and aids in assimilation of iron). and E (carries oxygen to the cells) are required. Calcium and magnesium, copper, iron and zinc are also needed.

Herbal Combinations: Anemia, blood purifier, digestion and liver.

Single Herbs: Key herbs are yellow dock (40 percent iron) and dandelion (helps the liver assimilate iron), alfalfa, kelp, dong quai and watercress. Also good are barberry, black walnut, burdock, cayenne, chaparral, echinacea, garlic, gentian (helps in digestion), ginger, goldenseal, hawthorn, lobelia, red clover and sarsaparilla.

Supplements: Beet powder (nourishes the blood), chlorophyll, blackstrap molasses, spirulina, evening primrose oil, blue-green algae.

Avoid: Coffee, black or green tea, white flour products, fried foods, excess fats and starches, excess protein, refined sugar, preservatives food and additives, canned foods, pasteurized milk.

✦ ANOREXIA NERVOSA AND BULIMIA

Anorexia nervosa and bulimia are eating disorders. Anorexia is a disorder mainly with young girls who starve themselves for thinness. One-third of those involved die. Bulimia is characterized by binge-eating then vomiting or using cathartics or diuretics. Starvation and purging are dangerous and will bring long-lasting health problems or even coma and death. Vomiting often leads to deterioration of the stomach and esophagus linings, an increase in cavities and gum disease and even the loss of teeth. It flushes essential minerals from the body which are necessary for proper metabolism and physical and mental well-being.

Extreme restriction on calorie intake can cause fluid and electrolyte disturbances leading to heart problems, kidney failure and urinary infections. It can lead to any auto-immune disease as well as lower the immune system for germs and viruses to take over.

The brain is also disturbed and can cause shrinkage of the brain mass in eating disorder victims. The body begins to cannibalize itself when it has no other source of nourishment. Muscle mass is depleted and the heart muscle can atrophy.

❖

Natural Therapy: Herbs are necessary to improve digestion, and strengthen the nervous system and glandular system. Education on the importance of good nutrition has to be stressed. People need to understand that the lack of minerals, especially zinc and potassium, can put a strain on the heart as well as other organs. When depleted through vomiting, low levels of copper can cause many body dysfunctions. All minerals are essential and when lost from the body cause destruction of the cells and organs.

Foods to Heal: Foods high in copper are leeks, garlic, artichoke, parsley beet root, dandelion greens and broccoli. The following foods are high in minerals: almonds, whole grains, molasses, egg yolks, green leafy vegetables, apricots and black figs.

Vitamins and Minerals: Take a multivitamin and mineral supplement. Vitamins A, B-complex, C with bioflavonoids, D, and E are essential. Also necessary are calcium and magnesium, potassium, sodium and zinc, which is quickly lost during starvation.

Herbal Combinations: Digestion, glands, hypoglycemia, and nerves. Stress and immune formulas will fortify the system.

Single Herbs: Alfalfa (very rich in minerals), black cohosh (protects the female organs), black walnut (helps balance minerals), burdock (purifies the blood), catnip (relaxes the nerves), chamomile (rich in calcium and relaxing for the nerves), chaparral, dandelion (feeds and protects the liver), echinacea, ginger (calms the stomach and helps in digestion), ginseng (strengthens the whole body), gotu kola (feeds the brain), hops (rebuilds the nerves), ho-shou-wu, kelp, lady's slipper (healing for the brain), licorice (provides energy and balances hormones), lobelia, papaya, passionflower, peppermint, skullcap (rebuilds and nourish the nerves), red clover, wild yam, wood betony, and yellow dock.

Supplements: The following supplements are vital when the body has been stripped and depleted of essential nutrients: free-form amino acids, evening primrose oil, fish oil lipids, acidophilus, green drinks and salmon oil. Germanium and coenzyme Q_{10} supply oxygen to the cells while blue-green algae will build up the immune system. Liquid chlorophyll will help build and purify the blood, and a liquid mineral and herbal formula will help restore mineral imbalance.

Avoid: All processed food. It is essential to eat organic food high in vit-amins and minerals. Avoid caffeine, alcohol, tobacco and white sugar products—they all deplete more minerals from the body. Avoid meat as it is high in uric acid and fat.

✤ APPENDICITIS

Appendicitis is a disease of constipation and incomplete elimination. It is an autointoxication, a self-poisoning from poor elimination. The appendix is needed in the body to help clean the cells so the lymphatic system can do its job of filtering the toxins. Appendicitis is inflamma-tion of the vermiform appendix due to an obstruction. It can occur at any age. If the appendix ruptures or perforates, the infected contents spill into the abdominal cavity, causing peritonitis, which is a very dan-gerous complication of appendicitis.

The appendix is lymph tissue and the lymphatic system helps protect the body from infections. If the appendix is removed the natural immune system is impaired. The appendix and tonsils become inflamed from lymphatic system congestion. Removing the appendix or the ton-sils interferes with the body's ability to respond in a natural way to tem-porary toxic congestion.

Natural Therapy: Cleaning the bowels, the blood and the liver is impor-tant. A pure water fast with psyllium increases bulk. Potassium broths made with onions, celery, potatoes (peels) and parsley are beneficial. A fast using fresh lemons, pure maple syrup and cayenne pepper in pure water is also cleansing and healing to the body.

Foods to Heal: A high-fiber diet increases bulk, prevents retention and incomplete elimination of the bowels. High-fiber foods are whole grains such as barley buckwheat, millet, whole wheat, cornmeal, brown rice, beans and lentils, and vegetables such as cabbage, aspara-gus, carrots, green peas, spinach, onions, potatoes. Berries also have a high content of fiber. Use fresh green salads daily, using leaf lettuce, cabbage, carrots, broccoli and any fresh vegetables.

Vitamins and Minerals: Take vitamins A and C to fight infection and the minerals selenium and zinc for healing. A multivitamin and mineral supplement is also beneficial.

Herbal Combinations: Infection fighters, immune, nervous, liver and lower bowels.

Single Herbs: Aloe vera (acts as a laxative and is healing), burdock (blood cleanser), cayenne, chaparral (cleans deep in the cells), comfrey (healing for the mucous membranes), echinacea (cleans the lymphatics), garlic, goldenseal (will clean and purify the blood), kelp (supplies minerals for healing), myrrh, pau d'arco (cleans the blood and protects the liver), rose hips, slippery elm (healing and nourishing), and yellow dock (rich in iron).

Supplements: Aloe vera juice (internally), acidophilus, chlorophyll (to clean the blood), lecithin, blue-green algae.

Avoid: Too much meat, potatoes and gravy, and low-fiber foods. Stay away from sugar and white flour products, and avoid deep-fried food because fried oils cannot metabolize in the body.

✦ ARTERIOSCLEROSIS/ATHEROSCLEROSIS

Plaques and deposits of fatty elements on blood vessel walls contribute to this circulatory disorder. It can hinder the flow of blood, thus leading to high blood pressure, strokes and heart attacks. Arterio- and atherosclerosis are called the silent killers because of its slow buildup along the artery walls. The accumulation usually starts around the heart first, then the arteries. It is known that fatty streaks are found in the aorta (main artery of the body) of children in almost every country and it is believed that the fatty streaks are the precursors of plaques. This is caused from poor elimination and a dysfunction of the gall bladder and the liver.

The liver, under normal circumstances, can eliminate toxins from the body. But when the liver is overburdened with toxins from the bowels that have not completely eliminated, it has to try to detoxify excess poisons. The liver has to dump the excess poisons into the bile. This thickens the bile and clogs the gallbladder. Since the liver is responsible for dealing with cholesterol, it cannot filter it properly when it is overloaded.

Natural Therapy: Blood purification, cleaning the bowels and short fasts. Use herbal therapies for the circulation, glands and muscular systems.

Change the diet to high-fiber foods, fruits, and a lot of vegetables. Eat nuts, seeds and sprouts to obtain protein.

Foods to Heal: Garlic, onions, salmon, sardines, and cod (contains omega-3 oil). Eat food containing nucleic acids; they build cell energy to help retard deterioration of the arteries and help repair DNA and RNA. Foods that contain nucleic acids are: asparagus, beets, whole grains, chick peas, kidney beans, honey, lentils, lima beans, millet, buckwheat, nuts, sardines, salmon, split peas, soy beans, tuna, and leafy vegetables.

Vitamins and Minerals: Take extra vitamin B6 and niacin, vitamin C with bioflavonoids, vitamin E (increases oxygen), choline, inositol (helps dissolve plaque), calcium, magnesium, chromium, selenium and zinc.

Herbal Combinations: Blood purifier, bone combination, heart, chelation, lower bowel formulas.

Single Herbs: Alfalfa, aloe vera (has a cleansing effect on the veins), black walnut, burdock, capsicum (equalizes blood circulation and cleans veins), chaparral (cleans deep in tissues), cascara sagrada (prevent toxins from accumulating in blood and cholesterol and prevents them from adhering to the walls of veins), comfrey, echinacea, garlic and parsley (work together to prevent plaque buildup), goldenseal, hawthorn (strengthens heart and supplies oxygen to blood), horsetail (supplies silicon, calcium and other minerals), juniper berries, Irish moss, kelp, licorice, marshmallow, pau d'arco, psyllium, red clover, slippery elm, watercress, and yellow dock.

Supplements: The amino acid alanine reduces cholesterol when combined with arginine and glycine. L-carnitine, cysteine, glutamine and methionine prevent accumulation of fat in the liver. Taurine, lecithin, evening primrose oil, salmon oil, coenzyme Q_{10}, fish oil lipids, germanium (lowers cholesterol), aloe vera juice and digestive enzymes are important for proper digestion.

Avoid: Red meat, white flour and sugar products, salt, high-fat foods, animal fats and shortening, fried foods, doughnuts, pastries, all deep-fat fried foods. Eliminate alcohol, caffeine, soft drinks, tea, white sugar, and white flour products. Do not become constipated as toxins can back-up into the bloodstream and cause other problems.

✤ ARTHRITIS (ALSO BURSITIS, GOUT, RHEUMATISM)

These disorders are characterized by inflammation of the joints. They can be caused by excessive calcium deposits, causing spurs or deposits of crystallized uric acids in the joints that irritate and cause pain. Research indicates that many arthritic conditions can be allergy-related. Elimination of certain dietary elements may prove very helpful. Arthritis is aggravated by an accumulation of toxic waste in the body. Arthritic tendencies can also be inherited.

Rheumatoid arthritis is a chronic, inflammatory disorder causing stiffness, deformity and pain to joints and muscles. It is an auto-immune disease where the body attacks itself as if it is a threat to the body. It can affect the lungs, blood vessels, spleen, skin and muscles. Early signs can be fatigue, muscular aches and pains, stiffness in the joints, and swelling. Osteoarthritis is a wearing-away ailment. Cartilage in joints wastes away and calcium spurs may form on surfaces that have contact with bones.

Natural Therapy: Herbal therapy to treat the skeletal/muscular, circulatory, glandular, and nervous systems is beneficial. A basic alkaline diet is good because with these diseases the body becomes acidic and the cartilage in the joints begins to dissolve because of acid in the blood. Blood purification is indicated. Use cleansing diets, short juice fasts (carrot and celery), and regularly cleanse the bowels. Distilled water acts as a chelating agent. Minerals are vital; the best kind are found in herbs. An herbal liquid formula with minerals is also excellent.

Foods to Heal: Fresh vegetable juices, fresh fruits, whole grains, okra, sprouts, yogurt, blackstrap molasses, and cherries are especially healing. Red cherry juice (non-sweetened) eliminates uric acid. Whey powder, okra and celery are high in sodium and prevent and dissolve deposits in the joints. Include in the diet bean sprouts, onions, cabbage, avocado, parsley, watercress, endive, yellow corn meal, barley, steamed brown rice, wild rice, millet, winter squash, green salads and potato-peel broth.

Vitamins and Minerals: Take vitamins A, B-complex (extra B_6, B_{12}, niacin and pantothenic acid), vitamin E, calcium and magnesium (in an herbal calcium formula), selenium, silicon, manganese and zinc.

❖

Herbal Combinations: Blood purifier, bone combination, comfrey, pepsin, digestion, nerve, pain.

Single Herbs: Key herbs are alfalfa (helps ease pain and its mineral content helps maintain acid/alkaline balance), chaparral (cleans deep in the muscles and joints), comfrey (helps build new tissue), dandelion, devil's claw (reduces inflammation and heals), hydrangea (has cortisone-like properties), kelp (rich in minerals for healing), yucca (stimulates natural cortisone), aloe vera, Brigham tea, burdock, capsicum, dulse, garlic, parsley, papaya, saffron (helps the body utilize oils), red clover, watercress, and white willow (helps in pain).

Supplements: Use free-form amino acids: cystine (works with pantothenic acid in arthritis treatment), histidine (removes heavy metals) and phenylalanine (for pain). Distilled water, green drinks, juices (carrot and celery) are beneficial. Coenzyme Q_{10}, fish oil lipids, salmon oil, evening primrose oil, rice bran syrup, chinese essential oils, tea tree oil (external), and lecithin (helps control the chemical balance of the joints) should also be taken.

Avoid: Red meat, white flour, white sugar, salt, cola drinks, fried foods, pork, fats, heated oils, citrus fruit, nightshade family foods (tobacco, tomatoes, potatoes, green peppers, eggplant), dairy products, potato starch (in canned and packaged foods), and environmental pollutants. It is also important to avoid digestive disturbances; they lead to a loss of nutrients because of poor digestion and assimilation. Undigested food ferments in the intestinal tract and toxins can enter the blood stream.

❖ ASTHMA

Asthma is a chronic, usually allergic, condition which causes difficulty in breathing and wheezing due to mucus and inflammation in the lungs. The body is congested with toxins and excess mucus. When the bowels are congested the lungs try to eliminate.

The lungs are one of the organs of elimination. Breathing properly is essential to cleanse the body of toxins, as well as help the body utilize nutrients. Exercising in fresh air helps the lungs increase their ability to pump oxygen. The vessels and circulation are kept healthy by the blood vessels.

❖

Incomplete digestion, poor nutrition and autointoxication, along with free radicals and rancid fats, can result in particles of matter which gradually close the pores. The lungs then lose their elasticity.

Air pollution can cause and worsen respiratory illnesses, including asthma, bronchitis, and pneumonia. Fine particulate matter (toxins in the air), suppress the body's immune system and may even cause cancer. Ozone is a very serious pollutant that can cause permanent lung scarring and decreased pulmonary function. Carbon monoxide binds with hemoglobin in the blood system. This decreases the ability of the blood to transport oxygen and can result in dizziness, headaches and slowed reflexes. Prolonged exposure to carbon monoxide may cause arterial or heart disease.

Natural Therapy: Lower bowel cleansing would be the most beneficial. Read information on autointoxication. Herbal therapy cleans and strengthens the lungs. Short fasts, cleansing diets and a positive attitude will speed healing.

Foods to Heal: Green leafy vegetables, sprouts, whey, yogurt, okra, sunflower seeds, black beans, onions, garlic, honey, fresh fruits and vegetables, nuts, seeds, oatmeal, brown rice and whole grains.

Vitamins and Minerals: Vitamin A (50,000 units to heal), B-complex (strengthens the nervous system), extra B6 (necessary due to metabolism deficiency), B12, pantothenic acid, vitamin C with bioflavonoids, vitamin E, calcium (to rebuild and relax the nerves), magnesium, manganese, herbal potassium (helps control mucus production), selenium, and zinc.

Herbal Combinations: Allergies, digestion, lungs, nerves, lower bowels.

Single Herbs: Key herbs are capsicum (dissolves mucus), cascara sagrada (keeps the bowels clean), comfrey, fenugreek (dissolves mucus and contains natural dehydrating properties), garlic (clears congestion from the lungs), horseradish (healing for the lungs), and lobelia (calming and cleansing for the lung). Other herbs are slippery elm, alfalfa, aloe vera (soothing and healing for the lungs), bayberry, black cohosh, ephedra (bronchial dilator and decongestant), burdock, chaparral, chickweed, dandelion, echinacea, eyebright, ginseng, goldenseal (expectorant and soothes inflamed mucous membranes), gotu

❖

kola, horsetail, ho-shou-wu, licorice, marshmallow (relaxes bronchial tubes, removes hardened phlegm and soothes irritated tissues in the lungs), ma huang, mullein, oat straw, pau d'arco, red clover, rose hips, skullcap, valerian, white willow, wood betony, yarrow and yellow dock.

Supplements: Use free-form amino acids to build new tissues, specifically glutathione, histidine and isoleucine to regulate glands. Chlorophyll and lemon juice are beneficial, as are RNA-DNA foods such as sardines, spirulina, bee pollen, tincture of lobelia for emergency, evening primrose oil, fish oil lipids, and salmon oil.

Avoid: Salt, starches, milk, chocolate, eggs, sugar, white flour, red meats. MSG (monosodium glutamate), sulfites, preservatives, and food colorings are all suspected to contribute to asthma.

❖ ATHLETE'S FOOT

Athlete's foot is a fungus infection of the skin of the feet, mainly between the toes. The fungus thrives in warm and damp places and is commonly transmitted from person to person through towels and locker rooms or bathroom floors. The fungus spreads quickly when friendly bacteria in the body is destroyed by antibiotics, sugar diet, drugs, or radiation.

Natural Therapy: Purify the blood, cleanse the colon, and eat a balanced diet. Soak the feet in water with antifungal herbs, such as pau d'arco tea. Also drink pau d'arco tea, about six cups daily.

Foods to Heal: Pure water, fresh fruits and vegetables, whole grains, yogurt (unsweetened), and garlic. Lemon juice and tea tree oil on the infected area is beneficial.

Vitamins and Minerals: Take vitamins A and C for healing the tissues and to stimulate the immune system. B-complex vitamins (yeast free), selenium (strengthens the immune system) and zinc (heals skin problems) are also beneficial.

Herbal Combinations: Blood purifier, candida formulas, cleansing, immune, nerve and stress combinations.

Single Herbs: Key herbs are black walnut (extract used externally will kill fungus infections), chaparral (antiseptic), echinacea (natural antibiot-

❖

ic), garlic (antibiotic), pau d'arco (blood cleanser) and red clover. Other herbs are alfalfa, capsicum, dandelion, dong quai, hops, horsetail (contains silicon and calcium to heal skin problems), kelp, lady's slipper, licorice, mistletoe, passionflower, sarsaparilla, skullcap, valerian, white oak (use externally as an antiseptic) and yellow dock (rich in iron for healing).

Supplements: Acidophilus, liquid chlorophyll, caprylic acid, salmon oil, evening primrose oil, tea tree oil (external use).

Avoid: Meat, sugar products of all kinds, salt, and white flour products.

❖ AUTISM

Autism is a type of mental illness which causes a person to withdraw into a private fantasy world and losing their ability to communicate with others in a real environment. Autistic people are not responsive to love and affection. Some of the children have low IQs but many are above average.

Natural Therapy: Blood purification, bowel cleaning, and brain and nervous system stimulation are beneficial. Make sure natural foods are given to autistic individuals. Nutrition is very important. The B-complex vitamins with extra B6 and magnesium have produced good results. Eliminate food colorings and preservatives from the diet.

Foods to Heal: Fresh fruit and vegetables, sprouts, whole grains (cooked in thermos), brown rice, millet, buckwheat, whole oats.

Vitamins and Minerals: Vitamin A builds the immune system, B-complex vitamins are essential for normal brain and nervous system function, and extra B6 deficiency has been linked to autism. Also take vitamin C with bioflavonoids and vitamin E. All minerals are important for brain function. Magnesium calms the nerves. Iron increases resistance to stress and disease. Selenium builds the immune system and retards formation of free radicals. Silicon is essential for all connective tissue health. Zinc is needed in the brain and nervous system.

Herbal Combinations: Blood purification, bowels, circulation, and the nerves.

Single Herbs: Key herbs are gotu kola, ginkgo (increases circulation), hawthorn, capsicum, lady's slipper (good for brain function), alfalfa, black walnut, dandelion, echinacea (blood cleanser), garlic, hops, licorice, lobelia, red clover, skullcap (strengthens nerves), wood betony.

Supplements: Evening primrose oil, salmon oil, spirulina, bee pollen, rice bran syrup, blue-green algae.

Avoid: All processed food, sugar, white flour products, caffeine, soft drinks, candy, chocolate, cake, cookies, pastries. Check for heavy metal accumulation.

✣ BACKACHE

Pain is the way the body tells you something is wrong, that you need to be aware of a certain area in the body. Aches are not as serious as pain and there are many different levels of aches and pains. Lower back pain can originate from constipation. Chiropractic treatments along with nutritional knowledge have helped many people cure their aches and pains. Headaches can also be caused by constipation and digestion problems. Stress can cause weakness in the body and create pain. Anger, frustration, grief, severe disappointment and anxiety can create pain in a weak spot in our body. People in poor health usually have aches and pains.

Are pain killers the answer? Americans spend millions of dollars each year on pain relievers. These pain pills usually give moderate relief with exposure to possible serious side effects. Ibuprofen has been known to cause liver cells to die. There have been thousands of reported cases of liver damage caused by acetaminophen listed in scientific literature. This is a drug that relieves pain and reduces fever. This drug can also cause kidney damage and encourage the formation of scar tissue in kidney cells. The best method in dealing with aches and pains is to prevent them through a healthier lifestyle.

Natural Therapy: Clean the lower bowels, purify the blood, strengthen the nerves, bones and muscles. Chiropractor adjustments are very beneficial. The bulk of the diet should consist of live foods.

Foods to Heal: Whole grains (cooked in thermos to protect live enzymes), sprouts, fresh vegetables and fruit. Take calcium foods such as sesame seeds, kelp, irish moss, dulse, collard leaves, kale, turnip greens,

❖

almonds, parsley, watercress, chickpeas, beans, sunflower seeds, okra, and endive.

Vitamins and Minerals: Vitamin C, iron and manganese are essential for production of new collagen. Calcium is needed (herbal is better). Zinc is necessary to maintain all tissues. Protein assimilation is essential.

Herbal Combinations: Bone, digestion, lower bowels, nerves, pain.

Single Herbs: Key herbs are comfrey (builds new tissues), horsetail, (contains calcium and minerals for healing) oatstraw, and slippery elm (rich in protein and healing properties). Other herbs are alfalfa (rich in minerals), aloe vera, burdock, dandelion, hops (relaxing), lady's slipper, skullcap (strengthens the nerves and helps pain) and white willow (pain reliever).

Supplements: Herbal creams for pain (external), chinese essential oils, peppermint oil, wintergreen oil.

Avoid: Heavy meat diet, constipation, drugs such as cortisone (destroys bones), bending forward without bending the knees. Also avoid lifting heavy objects. A heavy purse may injure the neck, shoulders and back.

❖ BEDWETTING

Bedwetting can be a concern for parents, but they should be patient with the child. A child cannot help the bedwetting and should not be scolded or punished. Allergies have been implicated in bedwetting. In fact, it has been seen in children where there is a family history of allergies or hayfever. Constipation can cause bedwetting since it puts pressure on the bladder. Bedwetting may be caused by emotional upsets, infections, or extreme fatigue (allergies can cause fatigue).

Natural Therapy: Purifying the blood and strengthening the urinary tract. Using food and herbs to strengthen the bladder, kidneys and the nervous system.

Foods to Heal: Foods high in calcium and magnesium are beneficial. Magnesium foods are kelp, almonds, cashews, soybeans (milk), dulse, sesame seeds, beans, millet, grains, and wild rice. Calcium foods are sesame seeds, kelp, irish moss, dulse, collard greens, kale leaves, almonds, soybeans, parsley, watercress, sunflower seeds, broccoli.

Vitamins and Minerals: Take a multivitamin and mineral supplement. Extra calcium and magnesium in an herbal formula is recommended. Silicon, manganese and zinc will strengthen the bladder.

Herbal Combinations: Bladder and kidneys, bone combinations, glands and nerves.

Single Herbs: Key herbs are buchu (heals and strengthens the bladder), cornsilk (cleans mucous membranes and heals), oatstraw (antiseptic properties), and uva ursi (cleans urinary tract). Other herbs that help are dandelion, hops, marshmallow (soothing and healing), parsley, (natural diuretic), skullcap, slippery elm (healing and nourishing) and St. John's wort.

Supplements: Bee pollen, evening primrose oil, salmon oil, chlorophyll.

Avoid: Foods involved in allergies: milk, chocolate, eggs, cereals, bread, corn, citrus fruits (unripened), food additives and colorings, carbonated and caffeine drinks. Avoid drinks before bed. Give nervine herbs during the day.

✤ BLADDER AND KIDNEY INFECTIONS

Cystitis is an inflammation of the bladder and is usually caused by bacteria. Kidney infections can result and are more serious. Frequent urination, pain, burning discomfort and a dark-colored and scanty urine can be symptoms. Backache and fever can occur in young children in addition to vomiting, nausea and diarrhea. The main cause is toxemia with impure blood and too many sweet foods causing an overly acid condition.

The kidneys have the job of filtering waste products from the blood. The kidneys also regulate the fluid and electrolyte balance in the body. The bladder holds the urine and if toxins accumulate without being eliminated often, it can develop infections. Drinking plenty of pure water will help keep the bladder clean.

Autointoxication is one cause of bladder and kidney infections. Constipation causes a back-up in the bloodstream which irritates the bladder and causes irritations. Congested kidneys will cause the skin to try and eliminate. The skin is the largest elimination organ of the body and takes over if the kidneys are plugged up with mucus material and toxins.

❖

The liver helps to detoxify and clean the blood and convert toxins into water soluble particles. The kidneys are the filters that collect toxic particles and pass them out of the body.

Natural Therapy: Blood purification, demulcent, antibiotic and antiseptic therapies. Juice fasting will help heal the kidneys and bladder. Liquid chlorophyll will purify the blood, pure apple juice, green drinks and citrus juices will cleanse and heal. Enemas or lower bowel cleansers in herbal formulas will also help eliminate toxins from the system.

Foods to Heal: Garlic, onions, potassium broths (potato peelings, carrots tops, parsley, celery, etc.), unsweetened cherry and cranberry juices (inhibit bacterial growth) and fresh lemon juice in pure water.

Vitamins and Minerals: Vitamin A, vitamin B-complex (extra B$_6$, pantothenic acid, choline), vitamin C with bioflavonoids, vitamin E, calcium and magnesium, manganese, potassium, selenium, and zinc. Magnesium and vitamin D help to dissolve calcium deposits.

Herbal Combinations: Bladder and kidney, digestion, infections, glands.

Single Herbs: Key herbs are cornsilk (strengthens and heals), garlic (natural antibiotic), hydrangea (natural diuretic to clean the the kidneys), juniper berries (natural diuretic) parsley (diuretic), and uva ursi (strengthens and tones the urinary system). Other herbs are alfalfa, burdock, dandelion, goldenseal (cleans and heals the urinary tract), kelp, marshmallow (soothing and healing), pau d'arco (cleans the blood), red raspberry, rose hips (rich in vitamin C for healing), yarrow.

Supplements: Liquid chlorophyll, acidophilus, flaxseed tea, and two amino acids: L-cysteine, and L-methionine.

Avoid: Carbonated beverages, tea, coffee, alcohol and caffeine soft drinks. Avoid sugar—it encourages infections. Avoid underwear which prevents air circulation (cotton is best). Toilet tissue should be used from the front to the back to prevent irritations and infections. Avoid constipation, this can cause irritations from a toxic buildup in the blood. Avoid a high milk diet; milk is rich in protein which will produce an acid condition. It is important to also avoid aspirin. Researchers at the Oregon Health Sciences University in Portland said there is no doubt that aspirin, taken over a long period of time in a cumulative dose of more than two kilograms, can cause permanent kidney damage requiring dialysis or transplants. Three tablets a day for three years could yield harmful dosages.

✤ Blood Poisoning (Gangrene, Tetanus)

Blood poisoning causes the blood to become infected and congested. This contamination can be carried to any part of the body. This occurs when the blood is contains too much acid and congested with toxins. It is considered toxemia of the blood. When a red streak appears, it can be very serious and a natural practitioner should be consulted.

Autointoxication is one cause of impure blood. This is a self-poisoning by way of the large colon. When constipation or incomplete elimination is present this will cause a back-up into the bloodstream. This can happen even if you have three bowel movements a day if the colon doesn't completely eliminate. This is caused by eating junk food, white flour products, pasta, spaghetti, macaroni, and dairy products.

Natural Therapy: Blood purification. Use teas of echinacea, pau d'arco, or red clover. These will enter the bloodstream and clean and purify the blood. A juice fast will also clean and build up the blood. Citrus juices will also cleanse. External therapies include plantain poultices, clay packs, black walnut and slippery elm.

Foods to Heal: Beets and beet greens, Swiss chard, alfalfa sprouts, parsley, cherries, grapes. Green drinks will help clean the blood. Blackstrap molasses is rich in iron and copper.

Vitamins and Minerals: Vitamin A (100,00 units for a while), vitamin C, every hour (watch for diarrhea, tolerance level) B-complex vitamins are involved with healing, especially B_{12} and folic acid (essential for the formation of healthy blood cells in the bone marrow). Selenium and zinc are healing. Vitamins C and E aid in the assimilation of organic iron. Iron obtained from yellow dock is natural. Copper transports nutrient-bearing oxygen to all parts of the body.

Herbal Combinations: Blood purifier, bone combination, immune formula, liver and gallbladder, lower bowel.

Single Herbs: Key herbs are burdock (one of the greatest blood cleansers),

❖

chaparral (cleans blood and cells), echinacea (lymphatic and blood cleanser), garlic (cleans and purifies the blood), goldenseal (cleans and purifies the digestive tract), pau d'arco (liver and blood purifier), and yellow dock (rich in organic iron). Other important herbs are alfalfa (rich in minerals), bayberry, black walnut (kills parasites and worms), butcher's broom, cascara sagrada (keeps the bowels regular), dandelion (liver cleanser), fenugreek (loosens hard mucus), kelp (cleans and nourishes the blood), licorice, sarsaparilla and yarrow.

Supplements: Blue-green algae, liquid chlorophyll, barley juice, lecithin, hydrochloric acid (insufficient will prevent the absorption of iron), and wheat grass juice.

Avoid: Junk food; it contributes to toxic blood. Avoid a low-fiber diet and constipation. Avoid alcohol, drugs, vaccinations (contain toxins and viruses), and all sugar products (leach nutrients from the body). A diet high in fat and meat will contribute to toxic blood.

❖ BRONCHITIS

Bronchitis is a general term used to describe inflammation of the mucous membranes inside the bronchial tubes. The lubricating glands of the bronchi become enlarged and the tiny hairs become clogged with mucus and is cleared by coughing. The air chambers can become strained and weakened. Coughing can linger as long as three months after an acute attack of bronchitis.

Bronchitis can be caused by polluted air or smoking which weakens the lungs. Allergies are often associated with bronchitis. When the body is strengthened and the mucous membranes cleaned of toxins, however, both allergies and bronchitis will clear up. Constipation or incomplete elimination of the bowels are also connected with bronchitis. The lungs are one of the organs of elimination and when the colon is congested it can back-up into the lungs.

Natural Therapy: Juice fasting along with enemas or bowel cleanser. The body becomes toxic from too many acid foods. An alkaline diet after cleansing the body will build up the lungs. Exercise will also build up the lungs and will help protect from infections.

Foods to Heal: Correct food combining will help heal the lungs while incomplete digestion and poor nutrition can irritate them. Citrus juices (tree ripened if possible) are also helpful. Frozen juices are second best if fruits are picked ripe and frozen. The diet should also include more alkaline foods and more fresh, raw fruits and vegetables. Salads using several kinds of leafy lettuce and vegetables. Barley water with lemon juice contains hordenine which relieves bronchial spasms. Unsweetened cranberry juice acts as an antiseptic.

Vitamins and Minerals: Vitamin A (up to 100,000 I.U.), fish liver oils, beta carotene, B-complex (speeds healing), and vitamin C with bioflavonoids, (large amounts to start). Vitamins D and E will also heal. Use a multimineral and take extra iron (found in yellow dock and dandelion), manganese, silicon, sodium and zinc.

Herbal Combinations: Allergy, blood cleansers, digestion, lower bowels, lungs, nerves.

Single Herbs: Key herbs are boneset (helps aches), cascara sagrada, comfrey, garlic (antiseptic), ginger, lobelia (chest constrictor), marshmallow (soothing and healing), mullein (heals lungs), and slippery elm (supplies protein and heals). Also helpful are capsicum, echinacea, goldenseal, eucalyptus, licorice, ma huang and pau d'arco.

Supplements: Hot lemon juice with ginger, liquid chlorophyll, royal jelly, bee propolis, blue-green algae.

Avoid: Too much intake of starchy foods, salt, sugar and meat. Cheese, fried foods, chocolate, pastries, refined cereals and pastas should also be avoided.

✤ BRUISING

Bruising is bleeding under the skin. The underlying tissues are injured, which results in swelling, black and blue marks and pain. Increased bruising may be a result of anemia, malnutrition, overweight, and/or lack of vitamins and minerals. High medication intake—aspirin for example—can also cause bruising.

Natural Therapy: Blood building therapy and a cleansing diet will help bruising. Eliminate acid-forming foods and add more alkaline foods to the diet. Cleansing the blood is important, for bruising can be a warning sign of cancer.

❖

Foods to Heal: Carrots, apricots, kale, spinach, collard greens, Swiss chard, beet greens, sprouts, wheat grass juice, grains (thermos cooking), chives, onions and garlic. Sesame seeds contain vitamin T which helps build healthy blood platelets.

Vitamins and Minerals: Vitamins A, C (with bioflavonoids), and K. Take a multimineral with extra selenium and zinc.

Herbal Combinations: Blood cleanser, bone, digestion.

Single Herbs: Key herbs are alfalfa, horsetail (strengthens bones, flesh and cartilage), kelp (healing and nourishing), rose hips (contains vitamin C and B-complex), slippery elm (heals skin), and yellow dock (rich in iron and minerals). Other herbs to help are black walnut, capsicum, dandelion, dong quai (blood builder), ginger, hawthorn, hops, lady's slipper, lobelia, marshmallow, skullcap, St. John's wort, and white oak bark (heals skin).

Supplements: Poultice of comfrey and black walnut mixed with aloe vera juice or pure water; liquid chlorophyll, essential fatty acids, redmond clay (externally), and blue-green algae.

Avoid: Smoking (depletes vitamin C), drugs, aspirin, refined foods, and caffeine (depletes minerals from the body). Anticlotting drugs can cause vessel rupture and thrombosis.

❖ BURNS

Tissues are damaged from burns caused by heat, hot water, electricity, chemicals (acid or alkaline), or radiation. They can range from a mild burn to charring and destruction of the skin. There are three basic types of burns: first-degree burns, which cause redness and some pain; second-degree burns, which cause redness and blisters; and third-degree burns, which cause destruction of the skin and underlying muscles. The first positive action in treating burns is to apply cold water (not ice water). Injury to the skin can be prevented if cold water is applied immediately.

Natural Therapy: First, treat the burn with cold water (apply until pain has stopped). If it is from an acid or chemical, flush the burn with water under the faucet to remove the irritating substance. First-degree burns can be treated with comfrey salves, aloe vera and vitamin E.

❖

Second-degree burns can be treated with a paste made from comfrey, honey and wheat germ oil. Vitamin E can be used on a healed burn to prevent scarring. Third-degree burns can be treated with the comfrey paste, honey and wheat germ oil. It is beneficial to have a live aloe vera plant in the house and use it for emergencies.

Foods to Heal: Almost all fresh green vegetables, freshly ground whole grains, cold-pressed vegetable oils, bananas, green peas, oats, corn, raw fruits, sweet potatoes, egg yolks. Extra protein is needed, (soy protein drinks), and also a lot of liquids, especially pure water.

Vitamins and Minerals: Vitamin A (100,000 I.U. daily for a while), vitamin C (with bioflavonoids), vitamin B-complex (extra B$_{12}$), and vitamin E (used both internally and externally). A multimineral supplement is important because burns heal faster when minerals are present. Also take extra calcium and magnesium, potassium, sodium, selenium, copper, and zinc.

Herbal Combinations: Bone (increases healing), infections, nerve and relaxant combinations. Lower bowel cleansers will help prevent infections.

Single Herbs: Aloe vera (very healing), chickweed (will purify the blood), comfrey (heals and restores damaged tissues), garlic, horsetail (contains silicon), marshmallow (for acid or fire burns), oatstraw, red clover, slippery elm (internal and external), witch hazel and yarrow.

Supplements: Aloe vera juice (decreases bacterial infections and speeds healing), evening primrose oil, salmon oil, chinese essential oils (used externally), redmond clay (make a paste), and tea tree oil (external).

Avoid: A high-sugar diet, sweet drinks, cortisone creams, ice water and acid foods (accumulate too many toxins in the body). Do not use butter or margarine on the burn—it will cause the burn to penetrate deeper.

❖ CANCER

There are many different types of cancer. Some spread quickly and others take years to develop. The bloodstream and the lymphatic system can take cancer cells to different parts of the body. Cancer is a severe disorder of the immune system where the replication processes of the cells malfunctions, causing cells to reproduce wildly and invade other organs and tissues. This is known as malignancy.

The basic causes of cancer are environmental, dietary and stress factors that allow normal cells to get out of control. Cancer is a risk all of us take because we cannot be at a well level all the time. Air pollution, pesticides, food additives and drugs all contribute to the degree of health we can maintain at any one time.

Natural Therapy: Blood purification and nervine therapy are important. The nervine herbs help strengthen the nervous system, which is connected to the immune system. When the nerves are strong and healthy the body can handle diet changes. The National Academy of Sciences validated what many nutritionally-oriented physicians have been saying for years—there is a connection between diet and cancer.

Foods to Heal: A change of diet is necessary. Cruciferous vegetables (cabbage, broccoli, bok choy, Brussels sprouts, cauliflower, cress, kale, mustard, horseradish, turnip, rutabaga and kohlrabi) protect against cancer. Scientific studies have discovered that these crucifers contain compounds called indol-3-carbinol that inactivates estrogen. Excess estrogen has been shown to promote the development of certain cancerous breast tumors, and diets high in cruciferous vegetables can decrease the risk of developing the disease. High-fiber diets will also protect against cancer. Foods rich in potassium: beans (sprouts first), whole grains (best sprouted), wheat grass juice, almonds, sunflower and sesame seeds, lentils, parsley, blueberries, coconut, endive, leaf lettuce, oats (thermos cooking), potatoes (baked with skin), carrots, peaches, fresh fruits and vegetables. Buckwheat, brown rice and millet (easy to digest and assimilate).

Vitamins and Minerals: Vitamin A (protects against bladder cancer) and B-complex vitamins (fortify the nerves). Vitamin C with bioflavonoids protects against all cancers. It works as an antioxidant, destroys, neutralizes and protects against additives, and detoxifies viruses and carcinogens which cause cancer. Vitamin D helps the body to use calcium, vitamin A and minerals. Vitamin E is a free-radical scavenger (works with selenium). It is also beneficial to take a multimineral with extra calcium, magnesium, magnesium, selenium, silicon and zinc.

Herbal Combinations: Blood purifier, bone, candida, cleansing, digestion, general cleanser, glands, immune, lower bowels, nerves.

Single Herbs: Key herbs are burdock (blood cleanser), garlic (natural antibiotic), capsicum (cleans the blood), chaparral (cleans the blood and eliminates toxins), echinacea (blood cleanser), kelp (cleans and nourishes the blood), lady's slipper, pau d'arco (protects the liver and cleans the blood), red clover (cleans the blood), and suma (strengthens the whole body).

Supplements: Acidophilus, liquid chlorophyll, blue-green algae, salmon oil and evening primrose oil, herbal teas containing red clover and chaparral, and pau d'arco tea.

Avoid: Refined grains and sugars, fried foods, and additives. Stay away from food colorings, coffee, tea, cola drinks. Avoid meat and eliminate salt-cured, salt-pickled and smoked foods such as sausage, bacon, ham, smoked fish, bologna and hot dogs. A high-fat and meat diet can cause colon cancer. Fluoride in water and toothpaste is linked to bone cancer. Obesity increases risk of colon cancer. Smoking causes lung and mouth cancer.

✢ CANDIDA (ALSO THRUSH)

Candida is a parasite which thrives in warm-blooded animals. It is scientifically classified as a fungus. This fungus can cause thrush and vaginal infections as well as spread to any part of the body that is weakened. The overgrowth of the fungus *Candida Albicans* is known as candidiasis. It debilitates the immune system and to get it under control, a person must adhere to a strict dietary regimen.

Candida multiplies and develops toxins which circulate in the bloodstream and cause all kinds of symptoms and illnesses. It causes chemical reactions in the body and can produce false estrogen, making the body think it has enough so that estrogen production slows down. It also deceives the body into thinking it has more than enough of the thyroxine, a thyroid hormone. These results can cause menstrual irregularities and hypothyroid problems.

Natural Therapy: Cleansing the blood, the lower bowels, and improving digestion and liver function is crucial. Antibiotics are the main cause of candidiasis because they destroy friendly bacteria. A change in diet will pay off in the long run.

❖

Foods to Heal: Focus on natural foods. Eat all vegetables—asparagus, broccoli, cabbage, greens of all kinds, cucumbers, peppers, lettuce, okra, beans, turnips, rutabagas, squash and potatoes. Onions, garlic, brussels sprouts, and kohlrabi are also good. Millet, brown rice, buckwheat, quinoa, amaranth are excellent grains. Unrefined oils such as safflower, soy, and olive oil should be used. Fiber is important for cleansing the intestinal tract as well as absorb toxins.

Vitamins and Minerals: Take a multivitamin and mineral. If it is natural and chelated it will be absorbed more easily. Vitamin A heals and B-complex strengthens the nerves. (Make sure the supplements you take are high potency and yeast free.) Vitamin C flushes the cells and heals. Calcium and magnesium balance. Take them with vitamin C, kelp and hydrochloric acid for better assimilation, Vitamin E increases body's resistance to stress and disease.

Herbal Combinations: Blood purifier, candida combination (with caprylic acid), cleansing (cleans cells), immune, nervine, stress.

Single Herbs: Key herbs are black walnut (kills parasites and fungus), burdock (purifies blood), chaparral (cleans deep in tissues), dong quai (blood purifier), echinacea (cleans lymphatics and blood), garlic (antibiotic), licorice, pau d'arco (kills fungus), red clover (purifies the blood), and white oak. Other herbs are alfalfa, capsicum, dandelion, hops, horsetail, kelp, mistletoe, passionflower, sarsaparilla, skullcap, valerian, and yellow dock.

Supplements: Acidophilus, evening primrose oil, salmon oil, caprylic acid, psyllium hulls.

Avoid: Antibiotic therapy, birth control pills, cortisone, progesterone suppositories, altered acid/alkaline balance, meat, high mercury levels, aspirin, chlorine in water, chocolate, fluoride, sleeping pills, nitrates/nitrites, and stress.

❖ CARDIOVASCULAR DISORDERS

Heart disease, stroke and related disorders kill more Americans than all other causes of death combined. Heart attacks will strike and kill over 60,000 Americans this year.

The heart accumulates fatty material around it before it accumulates on the veins; therefore it is usually advanced before you know you have heart trouble. Preventive measures can be taken before the heart is in serious trouble. One of the main causes, in my opinion, is constipation. The bowels back up and the liver cannot eliminate fatty material and it accumulates in the blood and on the arteries.

Natural Therapy: Blood purification, bowel cleansing and liver stimulation are excellent therapies. Focus on natural foods and eat a high-fiber diet. Exercise will strengthen the lungs and heart.

Foods to Heal: Whole grains are high in fiber and contain enzymes and B vitamins. Cook them in a thermos overnight. Raw fruit and vegetables, sprouts (live enzymes), asparagus, apples, bananas, beans, buckwheat (strengthens veins), seeds and nuts, whey powder, yogurt are also healing.

Vitamins and Minerals: Vitamins A, B-complex (extra B_3, B_6, B_{12}), E (increases oxygen in blood), and C with bioflavonoids (cleans and strengthens the veins). Also use pangamic acid, calcium and magnesium, copper, chromium, potassium, selenium and zinc.

Herbal Combinations: Blood purifier, chelation, digestion, heart, lower bowel, potassium.

Single Herbs: Key herbs are hawthorn (feeds and protects the heart), capsicum (cleans and nourishes the veins), garlic (protects the veins), burdock (blood cleanser), butcher's broom (strengthens the veins), ginseng (protects the body), gotu kola (food for the brain, horsetail, mistletoe, parsley, and saffron (helps digest oils). Other herbs are black cohosh, lobelia, bugleweed, blessed thistle, cramp bark, dandelion, ephedra, hops, kelp, lily of the valley, oatstraw, passionflower, rose hips, skullcap, St. John's wort, valerian, wood betony and yarrow.

Supplements: Chlorophyll, lecithin, flaxseeds, evening primrose oil, fish oil lipids, salmon oil, blue-green algae, Co Q_{10}, germanium, glucomannan.

Avoid: Smoking, high-meat diet, sugar (too much), constipation, liver congestion, caffeine, drugs, obesity, a sedentary lifestyle.

❖ CARPAL TUNNEL SYNDROME

Carpal tunnel syndrome is a condition that occurs when the median nerve that runs through the carpal tunnel opening in the wrist gets pinched or pressured due to constant repetitive motions. It is seen in workers who perform repetitive tasks, such as painters, carpenters, typesetters, meat cutters, assembly line workers, musicians, computer workers, and grocery store clerks. Symptoms—which include pain, numbness, tingling, and weakness in the hand muscles—appear to be most severe at night. The pain will become so severe that it will awaken the sufferer.

Carpal tunnel syndrome is becoming more and more common with the advent of the information age, where workers are spending hours a day typing on their personal computers. Dr. Arnold Fox believes a low-fat diet will help because fatty deposits in the wrist seem to be the main cause. He has seen patients respond to diet change, but as always, prevention is more important than treating this syndrome.

Natural Therapy: Blood purification therapy, liver, and lower bowel cleanser. Chelation therapy has also helped many people.

Foods to Heal: Brown rice, whole grains, soybeans, lentils, sunflower seeds, salmon, tuna, avocados, beans, cashews, oats, turkey. Fresh fruits and vegetables, eaten raw or lightly steamed, are very beneficial.

Vitamins and Minerals: Vitamins A, B, C, D, and E should be taken because they all help nourish and clean the veins. Also supplement with calcium and magnesium, potassium, silicon, copper, chromium, and zinc.

Herbal Combinations: Blood purifier, chelation, digestion, heart, lower bowel, potassium.

Single Herbs: Key Herbs: capsicum, garlic (antibiotic), Bugleweed, burdock, butcher's broom, dandelion, ginkgo (improves circulation), gotu kola, hops, hawthorn (cleans veins), kelp, oatstraw (cleans veins), rose hips, saffron (helps the body utilize fats), suma. Other herbs are black cohosh, lobelia, blessed thistle, cramp bark, mistletoe, parsley, passionflower, skullcap, St. John's wort, valerian, wood betony, yarrow, yucca.

Supplements: lecithin, evening primrose oil, salmon oil, blue-green algae, L-Carnitine, Co Q$_{10}$, germanium.

Avoid: Smoking, high fat diets, constipation, stress, caffeine, chocolate, sugar products.

✤ CATARRH (MUCUS)

This is an over-production of mucus in the respiratory system. Some call it a "chronic" cold that is punctuated with a runny nose, sinus problems, hay fever, allergies, cough, colds, tonsillitis, or earaches. People with catarrhal conditions are susceptible to all kinds of diseases. Catarrh is caused by the consumption of too many carbohydrates, sugars, starches and milk. It is aggravated by constipation. It starts in the stomach and can spread to the sinuses, tonsils, nasal cavities, ears, throat, bronchi and lungs.

Natural elimination must follow or many diseases can develop because germs and viruses seek the toxic waste and catarrh. Symptoms of catarrh include "hacking cough", a dry throat, bad breath, itching ears, sore eyes, upset stomach, gas, shortness of breath, constipation or diarrhea.

Natural Therapy: Fasting using lemon water (lemon has astringent and antiseptic properties), citrus juices, herbs and vegetable broths. Rest and chiropractic adjustments speed circulation for healing. Enema using catnip tea is good for children as well as for adults. Use an herbal laxative tea before going to bed; it will also bring fevers down quickly.

Foods to Heal: Garlic, onions (soak in hot water and drink the juice). Vegetable broth with potato peelings, onions, parsley, garlic, celery, carrots and tops, chives, and watercress.

Vitamins and Minerals: Vitamin A (essential for healthy mucous membranes), B-complex vitamins (depleted in acute diseases). C with bioflavonoids (necessary to prevent and heal catarrh conditions). All minerals are needed to prevent catarrh conditions. Calcium and magnesium, builds blood and sustains nerves. Potassium, sodium, selenium and zinc.

Herbal Combinations: Allergy, comfrey and fenugreek (heals and breaks up mucus), cold and flu formulas, infection, lower bowel, nerves and potassium.

Single Herbs: Alfalfa-mint tea, boneset (relieves pain and fevers), capsicum, comfrey (heals respiratory infections), echinacea (cleansing and healing), elder flowers (cleans mucus), fenugreek (loosens hardened mucous), garlic (natural antibiotic), ginger (settles stomach), goldenseal (heals infections), licorice, lobelia (works with other herbs to heal), marshmallow (soothes and heals catarrh conditions), ma huang, mullein (heals lungs), passionflower (relaxes), peppermint (settles stomach), rose hips (rich in vitamin C and B-vitamins), and slippery elm (provides protein for healing and heals throat and coughs).

Supplements: Acidophilus, aloe vera juice, liquid chlorophyll, blue-green algae, liquid herbal and mineral supplement, germanium, coenzyme Q_{10}.

Avoid: Mucus-forming foods such as milk, cheese, meat, bread, sugar, white flour products, pastries. Also avoid poor food combinations, such as eating starches with protein, or sugar with starches or protein. It is also important to recognize that overeating interferes with proper digestion and assimilation. Another thing to do is learn how to cope with stress in your life.

✤ Celiac Disease (Gluten Intolerance)

Celiac disease involves a severe intolerance to gluten. It is a relatively uncommon disorder which can result from a genetic weakness or from environmental factors. One theory is that ingesting gluten may trigger a preexisting immunologic response in a genetically susceptible person. Another theory is that a person with celiac disease may have an enzyme defect that causes an inability to digest gluten. This results in tissue toxicity as well as damage and weakness to the surface membranes of the small bowel.

Symptoms of celiac disease may include diarrhea, large and frequently foul-smelling stools that float, anemia, skin rash, nausea, abdominal distention due to flatulence, stomach cramps, weakness and weight loss.

Natural Therapy: Prevent irritation by eliminating gluten foods from the diet. Wheat, barley, rye and oats are the highest in gluten. Read food labels carefully to be certain that they do not contain gluten. The intestinal lining of the small intestine does not have the ability to absorb essential nutrients and the loss of vital minerals and vitamins can cause serious problems.

❖

Foods to Heal: Carrots, apricots, sweet potatoes, sprouts, fertile eggs, yellow fruits and vegetables, raw goats milk, blackstrap molasses, legumes, green leafy vegetables, almonds, beans, root vegetables, sunflower seeds, berries, avocados, potatoes.

Vitamins and Minerals: Vitamins A, D, K and E may be deficient because of the body's inability to absorb fat. B-vitamins, C and iron are depleted quickly with diarrhea. All minerals must be supplemented, especially calcium and magnesium.

Herbal Combinations: Blood purifier, anemia, digestion, bone.

Single Herbs: Alfalfa, burdock (blood cleanser), dandelion, kelp, papaya, psyllium (cleans the pockets of the colon), saffron (helps digest oils), slippery elm (healing and high in protein), and yellow dock.

Supplements: Chlorophyll, blue-green algae, glucomannan (cleans colon), acidophilus, flaxseed tea, essential fatty acids.

Avoid: Wheat, oats, barley and rye. Stay away from sugar (it depletes nutrients) and white flour products. Avoid fried foods and too much oil.

❖ CHEMICAL IMBALANCE

"Chemical imbalance" describes any condition which changes normal body patterns or chemical reactions. It is not a specific disease, but it has been implicated in persons who are depressed and mentally disturbed.

A set of brain chemicals called neurotransmitters control our emotions. These may be unbalanced even when the rest of the body seems healthy. The brain is extremely sensitive. In autointoxication, the brain suffers extreme toxic effects when the body seems strong in some other areas, and this condition will alter the functions of neurotransmitters.

Evaluating nutritional requirements is necessary in order to understand what the body needs in the case of a chemical imbalance. A healthy liver is essential for a healthy brain as the liver is responsible for regulating hormones. It helps eliminate estradiol, the unfavorable type of estrogen. If estradiol is allowed to enter the bloodstream, it can travel to the brain and cause depression and bizarre mental manifestations. The one natural source to help chemical reactions in the brain is wholesome food. The brain is the seat of our emotions and is an organ of the body which needs nutrients just as much as the liver or heart.

❖

Intestinal toxemia cannot be overlooked in cases of depression, mental illness, or other types of brain dysfunction. In the early 1900s, many medical doctors diagnosed toxemia (self-poisoning) as the major cause of illness. Dr. Henry A. Cotton, a physician involved with performing autopsies on mentally ill patients, found that every body he examined had a colon with one or more problems. Colon problems result in bacterial poisons—poisons that eventually act on the nerve supply of the abdominal organs and cause spastic colitis. They also contribute to the atony and atrophy of bowel walls, resulting in delayed motility, constipation and stasis. The ileocecal valve soon ceases to function normally and ileal stasis follows.

Natural Therapy: In order to change the imbalance of the body, and to eliminate symptoms and to help the body heal itself, we need to activate chemical responses that adjust conditions back to a more desirable state of balance. Blood purification and lower bowel cleansing are necessary to eliminate the toxins from traveling to the brain. The nerves need to be fed and strengthened.

Foods to Heal: Thermos-cook whole grains to retain B-vitamins and enzymes. Millet, buckwheat, and brown rice are excellent foods. Raw and lightly steamed vegetables, fruits are health building. Eat sprouts and herbs to replace the elements that cause an imbalance.

Vitamins and Minerals: B-vitamins are essential for brain function. Vitamins A, C and E and the mineral selenium boost energy in the brain. Lecithin is necessary for proper brain function. All minerals are essential for proper body function.

Herbal Combinations: Blood purifiers, bone, digestion, immune, lower bowels, nerve, stress.

Single Herbs: Key herbs are ginkgo (an antioxidant and increases circulation in the brain), gotu kola (feeds and nourishes the brain), suma (provides oxygen to the brain), dong quai (blood cleanser), ginseng (fortifies the whole body), goldenseal (eliminates toxins), hops (strengthens the nerves), licorice (provides energy and feeds the glands), passionflower (relaxes nerves). Other beneficial herbs are alfalfa, black cohosh, black walnut, burdock, capsicum, chaparral, dandelion, ephedra, echinacea, garlic, ginger, hawthorn, ho-shou-wu,

❖

lady's slipper, lobelia, psyllium, red raspberry, red clover, sarsaparilla, skullcap and yellow dock.

Supplements: Bee pollen, spirulina, chlorophyll, evening primrose oil, salmon oil, coenzyme Q_{10}, germanium and blue-green algae.

Avoid: Constipation, caffeine drinks, smoking, alcohol, chocolate, sugar products. Eliminate fried foods as they cause free radicals which reduce immunity.

❖ CHEMICAL TOXICITY

Chemical additives and environmental toxins are a real health hazard. Our only defense is to strengthen our immune system. We need to be concerned about the water we drink, the food we eat and the air we breathe. Radioactive isotopes are invisible, odorless and tasteless, and radiation of any kind is cumulative. Strontium 90 is very prevalent. In fact, scientists say that everyone has potentially dangerous amounts of radioactive strontium in their bones. It can cause leukemia, sarcoma of the bones (bone cancer), Hodgkins disease, anemia, and weakness in the immune system.

One our greatest threats is plutonium, created from nuclear plants. We have tons of nuclear waste stored in the United States. This waste is blown in the air, dumped in the soil, and filters into our water. It can cause lung cancer, leukemia, lymphoma and myeloma and cancer of the testes and ovaries.

Herbicide and pesticide residue are everywhere. We are constantly being exposed, and residue is found in the blood of persons living in both urban and rural areas. These poisons are capable of causing mutations and cancer. Lindane (bug bombs) is one example of a dangerous pesticide. It is used in home gardens and on farms for fruits and vegetables, yet it is a highly hazardous product. It is also used to treat seeds and hardwood lumber, and is popular in animal shampoos, flea collars, shelf paper and floor wax. It can cause cancer, is toxic to a growing fetus, damaging to reproductive organs, toxic to fish, and children are very susceptible.

Chemical additives in our food are also numerous—the number of additives has tripled in the past twenty years. Americans eat about ten pounds of chemical food additives a year. They are put in seeds before they are planted, put on crops as they grow, and put on food as it is shipped to the consumer.

Natural Therapy: Learn to read labels. Frozen food has a large amount of preservatives and additives. Learn to demand organically grown food. Eat a balanced diet using more alkaline foods than acid. Keep the bowels in good working order and the bloodstream pure and clean.

Foods to Heal: Raw or lightly steamed vegetables. Vegetable salads using sprouts (alfalfa, radish, fenugreek) and other vegetables. Fruit is cleansing to the body. Eat whole grains cooked in a thermos or slow cooking in low heat to preserve enzymes. Beans are also a natural protection against built-up chemicals.

Vitamins and Minerals: Vitamins A, D and E protect the immune system. Vitamin C with bioflavonoids protects the veins and immune system. B-complex protects the nerves. Multiminerals with extra calcium, selenium and zinc are also necessary.

Herbal Combinations: Blood purifier, bone, chelation, digestion, immune, lower bowels, glands.

Single Herbs: Key herbs are bugleweed, chaparral (cleans and eliminates toxins), echinacea (blood cleanser), garlic (neutralizes acids), horseradish (antibiotic properties), kelp (attracts chemical and moves them out of the body), pau d'arco (cleans blood and protects liver), psyllium (cleans and removes toxins), red clover (blood purifier), and yellow dock. Other beneficial herbs are alfalfa, aloe vera, comfrey, fenugreek, horsetail, dulse, ginkgo and suma.

Supplements: Blue-green algae, chlorophyll, pectin and wheat grass. Hydrochloric acid is essential in the blood to fight chemicals, infections, worms and parasites, and to maintain the acid-alkaline balance. Salmon oil is also beneficial.

Avoid: Sugar—it is one cause of breaking down the immune system. The lungs breathe in chemicals so avoid sprays if possible. Avoid fried foods, a high-meat diet, refined starches, salt, and a high-fat diet.

✤ Childhood Diseases

Childhood diseases are the body's way of cleansing and healing the body from inherited or acquired weaknesses. Germs cannot exist in a

❖

healthy and clean body. Germs are nature's scavengers and can live only on weak cells, toxins in the body, and excess mucus. If a child has a good strong body, he or she will not get childhood diseases. But when children have access to sugar products and consume them daily, the body weakens, inviting germs to feed off the toxins. Sugar is a major culprit in a weakened American diet; it leaches the body of nutrients that are vital for health. Processed food is void of the minerals, vitamins and natural fiber essential for a healthy immune system.

Childhood diseases include chicken pox, measles, mumps, rubella (German measles), rheumatic fever, scarlet fever and whooping cough. Vaccinations are supposedly a protection from the usual childhood diseases, but children go on to suffer allergy-related (atopic) conditions. In England, researchers from Southampton General Hospital have discovered that measles may well prevent atopy. (*Lancet,* June 29, 1996).

During chicken pox, avoid aspirin because of its known implications in causing Reyes syndrome. Measles cause a skin rash, and can lead to complications such as pneumonia and other lung, ear and eye infections. Mumps is a contagious viral infection and can spread to the ovaries, pancreas, testicles and the nervous system. Rheumatic fever is a strep infection and can affect the brain, heart and joints. Scarlet fever is a strep infection with sore throat, swollen lymph glands and cough. Scarlatina is a mild form of scarlet fever.

Natural Therapy: Childhood diseases should be taken seriously and treated naturally. Keep the child warm and dry. Give plenty of liquids, especially citrus juices. Complications can follow childhood diseases if they are not treated properly. Vegetable broths will help and use plenty of pure water. For fever, sponging with cold tap water will help bring it down. Avoid bright lights. Be alert for warning signs such as a high fever, delirium, listlessness, chest pains and breathing problems.

Foods to Heal: Citrus juices diluted with pure water are cleansing and healing. Barley water with slippery elm bark will nourish and soothe the digestive tract, especially when diarrhea is present. Fasting is the best method so the liver can eliminate the toxins. Green drinks are cleansing, as is wheat grass juice.

❖

Vitamins and Minerals: Vitamin A is healing for the lungs and mucus membranes. Supplement with B-complex vitamins because they deplete quickly in illness. Vitamin C with bioflavonoids will heal and help eliminate the toxins. Minerals are depleted fast in fevers and illness, so five the child extra calcium and magnesium, potassium, selenium and zinc.

Herbal Combinations: Cold and flu combinations, blood purifier, bone (extra calcium and minerals), immune, insomnia and pain, lower bowel.

Single Herbs: Key herbs are catnip (acts as a sedative), chamomile (calming for the nerves), echinacea (cleans lymphatics and blood), elderflower (reduces fever along with peppermint), garlic (a natural antibiotic), ginger (soothes stomach cramps), goldenseal (very strong antibiotic, kills worms), hops (relaxes nerves), lobelia (relaxant and removes obstructions), mullein, pau d'arco (blood cleanser), peppermint (use after vomiting to calm stomach), red clover (blood cleanser), rose hips (rich in vitamin C and B-complex), slippery elm, yarrow. Other herbs are alfalfa, capsicum, cascara sagrada (cleans bowels), eyebright, lady's slipper, pleurisy root, red raspberry (soothing in fevers), safflower, skullcap and yellow dock.

Supplements: Chlorophyll, aloe vera juice, and instant vitamin-C drinks.

Avoid: Stop eating food. The liver and stomach are overburdened with eliminating the toxins and are unable to effectively digest food. Sweets, alcohol, tobacco, chocolate, meat, and any food that interferes with healing should be eliminated during the illness. Stay away from drugs because they overstimulate the body. And remember that natural healing takes time. Mother Nature cannot be rushed.

❖ CHRONIC FATIGUE SYNDROME

Research into post-polio syndrome and chronic fatigue has made the astounding discovery that the virus which most often triggers chronic fatigue syndrome is closely related to the one that causes polio (*What Doctors Don't Tell You,* January 1996). Chronic fatigue syndrome (CFS) seems to be an alternative polio. Some researchers say that CFS is just another form of polio that has increased with the advent of polio vaccination. It is estimated that one in every 500 Americans may have CFS, according to the Centers for Disease Control.

❖

Guillain-Barre Syndrome is also connected with CFS. "Many gut viruses other than polio virus 1-3 can cause paralytic polio and CFS. This is because they can attach to more than one set of tissue receptors found on different cells in the brain, spine and other body areas, as can polio. Injury to such cells results in CFS symptoms, which also occur in polio and post-polio syndromes" (Jones, 2).

CFS is more common in women than men. It strikes between the ages of twenty and forty. It is one of degenerative disorders, which are very common in the United States and other highly developed countries. Symptoms are extreme fatigue, sore throat, recurrent upper respiratory tract infections, swollen lymph nodes, aching joints and muscles, memory loss, headaches, irritability, deep depression, and poor concentration. Stress is also implicated in CFS, which weakens the immune system.

Deficiency of valuable nutrients can cause a breakdown in the immune system. Lack of nutrients allows germs, viruses, bacteria, worms and parasites to flourish. This weakens the immune system and the nervous system, and causes diseases such as CFS to weaken the body.

Natural Therapy: Blood purification to rid the body of toxins. Bowel cleansers to clean the entire digestive tract and make certain that nutrients can be absorbed and utilized with the addition of hydrochloric acid and digestive enzymes. Candida is usually involved when the immune system is weak. A candida diet would help restore natural flora to the system. This fungus can prevent the body from utilizing sugars properly, blocking the body's energy production and causing extreme fatigue. Nervine therapy is essential. The immune and nervous systems are connected and need to both be treated. Exercise is very beneficial. Reduce stress in life. Fresh air is necessary to protect the lungs and blood. If a person is strong, but has constipation problems they can go on fresh fruit and vegetables and juices, sprouted grains and seeds, vegetable broths, fresh wheat grass juice or powdered barley or wheat grass, chlorophyll, blue-green algae, and can use enemas or clonics. If a person is weak, he/she can build the body up first and then use stronger therapies.

Foods to Heal: Foods to nourish the immune system include brown rice, whole grains such as buckwheat, millet, whole oats, rye and yellow corn meal, fresh fruits and vegetables, sprouts, seeds, nut milks and vegetable juices. Vegetables such as broccoli, cabbage, cauliflower, brussels sprouts, parsley will also protect the immune system.

Vitamins and Minerals: Vitamin A increases resistance to infections and protects against pollution, cancer and viral infections. Vitamin E prevents the oxidized state that cancer cells thrive in. It deactivates the free-radicals that promote cellular damage leading to malignancy. Vitamin C with bioflavonoids can activate white blood cells to battle foreign substances and increase the production of interferon, the body's antivirus protein. B-complex vitamins are vital, protect the nervous system, prevent fatigue and increase resistance to disease. Take extra B_{12} to prevent anemia and increase energy. B_6 helps in absorption of B_{12} and in the production of hydrochloric acid. A multimineral supplement is necessary for proper composition of body fluids, in blood and bone formation, and in maintaing proper nerve function. They are essential for enzyme function. Selenium and zinc protect against cancer but they are lost in food processing. Zinc is also vital for the immune system. It produces histamine which dialates capillaries so that blood carrying immune-fighting white blood cells can hurry to the scene of an infection. Calcium helps prevent heavy metals from accumulating in the body. Magnesium produces properdin, a blood protein that fights invading viruses and bacteria. Manganese activates enzymes that work with vitamin C. Iodine, iron, and chrominum are also important.

Herbal Combinations: Lower bowel cleansers, blood purifiers, candida, nervine formulas, immune formulas, bone and cartilage formulas.

Single Herbs: The following herbs help stimulate interferon production in the body: kelp, dulse, blue-green algae, ginkgo, milk thistle, pau d'arco, schizandra, siberian ginseng, suma, dong quai, echinacea, red raspberry, and ho-shou-wu. Also beneficial are burdock and red clover (help to clean the blood), goldenseal (a great cleanser and healer), capsicum (cleans the veins), echinacea (lumphatic and blood cleanser), garlic (antibiotic properties), and licorice (enhances the glandular system). Skullcap, hops, valerian, St. John's wort, chamomile, passionflower all strengthen the nervous system.

Supplements: Acidophilus (restores friendly bacteria), bee pollen (rich in nutrients, protects against allergies), essential fatty acids(essential for overall health), Lecithin (strengthen the brain and myelin sheath), coenzyme Q_{10} (protects heart and brain), free-form amino acids (repairs tissues and organs), hydrochloric acid (breaks down protein, helps in assimilation of minerals), and digestive enzymes (needed to break up viruses, worms, parasites and undigested protein).

Avoid: Sugar, alcohol, mushrooms and all fungi, molds and yeast in any form, soy sauce, all dry roasted nuts, potato chips, soda pop, bacon, salt pork, lunch meats, hot dogs, fermented foods such as sauerkraut, cheeses of all kinds. Eliminate all processed foods and all white flour products.

✤ CIRCULATION PROBLEMS (COLD HANDS AND FEET)

The circulatory system consists of the heart, arteries, veins, and lymphatics. They serve as the body's transport system, bringing life-supporting oxygen and nutrients to cells, removing toxic waste, and carrying hormones from one part of the body to another. Poor circulation is seen in the extremities of the hands, fingers, feet, toes, the head, the nose and genitals. Poor circulation is felt by cold fingers and toes, cold nose, tingling feelings in the extremities, muscle aches, impotency in male, frigidity in the female, dry eyes (or any other mucous membrane), ringing of the ears, dizziness, irritability and insomnia.

Toxins can be a cause of poor circulation. The blood carries nutrients to all parts of the body, but it also can carry toxins to any organ or part of the body. Autointoxication can cause the blood to carry toxins that will accumulate in the veins and interfere with proper blood circulation. This can cause cold hands and feet. When the blood is overloaded with toxins, circulation becomes impaired. Insufficient supply of blood is seen in diabetes or when there is an accumulation of plaque on the inner lining of the blood vessels. Stress is another cause of poor circulation. When under stress the nervous system inhibits complete blood vessel dilation.

Natural Therapy: Blood purification and skin brushing along with hot and cold showers. Exercise will help increase circulation. Do deep breathing exercises and learn to control stress, a factor in the con-

❖

striction of vessels and poor circulation. A common-sense approach to circulatory problems would be to create a natural nutritional program to prevent further accumulation of plaque, to dissolve particles already present, and to clean the arteries of material to provide for better circulation.

Foods to Heal: Eat a high-fiber diet. Oat bran will help in circulation by lowering cholesterol levels. Include bananas, broccoli, brown rice, millet, beans, peas, and a lot of green salads with lots of raw vegetables in the diet. Citrus juices and vegetables juices such as carrot, beet, celery, parsley are also very good. Green vegetables are blood cleansers. Also take green drinks using wheat grass, sprouts, parsley, comfrey leaves.

Vitamins and Minerals: Vitamins A, D and E are essential for a healthy circulatory system. Niacinamide-niacin (deficiency can result in depression, sleeplessness, body aches and irritability), and B-complex vitamins increases circulation and reduces cholesterol levels. Vitamin B_6, removes excess water in the tissues (poor circulation can be due to water excess). Vitamin C with bioflavonoids are necessary for healthy veins, especially the capillaries. Choline and inositol (found in lecithin). Multimineral with extra selenium and zinc (helps in glandular problems, anemia and in insomnia). Magnesium along with vitamin D is necessary for calcium assimilation. It removed excess calcium from the blood stream.

Herbal Combinations: Blood purifier, chelation, digestion, heart, potassium.

Single Herbs: Key herbs are hawthorn (nourishes the heart and veins), capsicum (increases circulation and cleans the veins), lobelia, garlic (lowers cholesterol), bugleweed (equalizes circulation), burdock (a blood cleanser), butcher's broom (improves circulation to prevent blood clots), ephedra, ginkgo, ginseng, gotu kola (improves brain circulation), horsetail (strengthens the immune system), mistletoe (constricts blood vessels), parsley (natural diuretic), psyllium (cleans colon of toxins), prickly ash (increases circulation in cold extremities and joints), skullcap. Other herbs are black cohosh, blessed thistle, cramp bark, dandelion, hops, kelp, lily of the valley, oatstraw, passionflower, rose hips, saffron, St. John's wort, valerian, wood betony and yarrow.

Supplements: Chlorophyll (rebuilds heart), lecithin (prevents and dissolves fatty deposits), flaxseeds, evening primrose oil, fish oil lipids, salmon oil (dissolves fatty deposits in the blood), glucomannan, rice bran syrup, coenzyme Q1O, germanium, L-carnitine, apple pectin (lowers cholesterol and regulates bowel function).

Avoid: Coffee, tea, cola or other caffeinated beverages, alcoholic drinks, and smoking. All cause circulation problems. A high-meat diet produces uric acid, and toxins. Constipation will cause toxins to accumulate in the blood and create poor circulation. Avoid fatty and greasy foods, sugar, salt and hydrogenated oils. Fats clog up the lymphatic system and slow the natural eliminatory system.

✤ Colds, Flu and Fever

Colds, flu and fevers are part of nature's eliminative process, a safety valve which the body opens of its own accord to give the body the chance for a natural process to take place. If we use drugs to suppress the flu or colds, that which should have been eliminated is retained within the body. As long as we continue to suppress the natural process of elimination the toxic material begins to settle in the organs of the body to eventually create what we call chronic disease such as arthritis, diabetes, chronic asthma, etc.

Modern medical science's theory is to kill the germ and cure the disease. Drug therapies have been developed that suppresses the acute diseases which either complicates the condition or throws it deeper into the organs to cause a chronic disease later. All acute diseases are based on Nature's Law. Scientists all around the world have been seeking for a cure to eliminate the common cold. They will never find a cure for acute diseases, for the diseases are the cure.

Natural methods create a positive effect on the health of the whole body. If drugs are the method chosen to treat acute diseases, the body is hindered in its ability to eliminate the toxins and causes them to remain in the body usually in the weakest part. Fever speeds up the body's healing process. The heart beats faster, the liver increases its activity destroying more toxins, the kidney's excrete more acids to clean the blood, the glandular system produces more hormones for normal body function and the body cells produce more interferon to fight illness.

❖

Natural Therapy: Cleansing the colon and blood purification will help eliminate the toxins. Because the body is trying to eliminate toxins by dumping them into the stomach, it is helpful to not eat. When eating, the healing and cleansing has to stop so that food can digest. Use herbal teas and citrus juices for cleansing the body. A lot of rest is necessary for healing.

Foods to Heal: Citrus juices with herbal teas are the most healing. Vegetable broths will strengthen the system.

Vitamins and Minerals: Vitamin A heals and protects the immune system. Vitamin C (with bioflavonoids), heals and destroys germs and viruses. B-vitamins are needed during illness. A multimineral supplement is needed for all healing and to maintain nutritional balance. Selenium, zinc calcium and magnesium are healing. Potassium is lost during illness, so a supplement is necessary.

Herbal Combinations: Allergy, cold and flu, infection, lower bowel, nerves, and potassium.

Single Herbs: Alfalfa and mint tea, aloe vera, capsicum, comfrey dandelion, fenugreek, garlic, ginger (settles stomach), goldenseal, kelp (provides minerals and heals), licorice, lobelia, marshmallow, mullein, passionflower, red raspberry, rose hips, slippery elm (for coughs and to heal throat).

Supplements: Aloe vera juice, liquid chlorophyll, blue-green algae.

Avoid: Eating solid food, meat, grains, sugar, and sweet fruit juices until healing takes place.

❖ COLITIS (DIVERTICULOSIS)

Colitis is an inflammation of the colon which causes loose and watery stools, often containing mucus, diarrhea and bleeding from the rectum. There can be alternate constipation and diarrhea, incomplete emptying of the bowels, and pain. Other symptoms are indigestion, headaches, fatigue and distension. It is a disease of the large intestine and affects an estimated 250,000 people in the United States.

There are different types of colitis, which can be mild or serious. Inflammation of the small intestine such as enteritis and ileitis are associated with colitis. In severe cases there can be anemia, weight loss, fever and a tender, bloated stomach.

❖

Natural Therapy: Healing therapy using demulcent herbs can be effective. Enemas or colonics to clean the bowels are also good therapy. Use mild food until healing takes place. Nervine herbal therapy can speed healing. A change in diet and lifestyle will eventually stabilize peristaltic movements and remove irritation. Try to reduce worry, tension and fatigue as they can put a burden on the colon.

Foods to Heal: A few days of fasting using carrot juice and demulcent herb teas like comfrey, mullein and slippery elm is healing. Steamed carrots, potatoes, and squash; avocados, eggplant, and bananas; and grated fresh apples, pears and peaches are all healing foods. Avoid the skin of fruits and vegetables until healing takes place. Put steamed or raw vegetables into a blender. Add psyllium or oat bran to liquids.

Vitamins and Minerals: Vitamin A (heals mucous membranes), vitamin C and bioflavonoids (build the immune system), vitamin E for tissue healing, vitamin B-complex (necessary for health and digestion), mineral supplement (lost in diarrhea) also essential for healing. Also take calcium, magnesium, chromium, zinc, silicon and selenium. A deficiency of vitamins A, E, and K is common in colitis.

Herbal Combinations: Bone and potassium, ulcer, digestion and lower bowels. Nervine herbs help in all healing.

Single Herbs: Aloe vera (very healing), alfalfa (contains vitamin K), dandelion, garlic, hops, kelp, lobelia, marshmallow, myrrh, papaya, pau d'arco, psyllium, skullcap, slippery elm, yellow dock.

Supplements: Acidophilus (milk-free), liquid chlorophyll, salmon oil, or evening primrose oil, glucomannan (before meals), blue-green algae.

Avoid: Over-the-counter laxatives (only irritates more), sugar, and other refined carbohydrates, insufficient chewing of food. Avoid emotional conflicts. Stress is an aggravating factor in colitis. Avoid fried food, condiments and excessive amounts of dairy products, chocolate, and caffeine drinks. Avoid smoking, fumes and chemical sprays, and toxic food additives.

❖ CONSTIPATION

Lack of fiber in the American diet is the main cause of constipation. The lack of fiber causes the food to remain too long a time in the colon and causes bacteria and toxins to accumulate. The longer food is retained, more water is absorbed, leaving the waste material dry, hard and difficult to evacuate. Under normal conditions the colon produces mucus to protect the intestinal wall, which keeps the material moving at a regular and smooth pace. But with constipation the colon loses its natural mucus when the water is absorbed, and the feces attach themselves directly to the intestinal wall. This builds up over the years with a high fat and white flour diet which is like putting paste or glue-like substances on the colon walls. This creates chronic diseases and, unless it is eliminated, can cause cancer and other life threatening ailments.

Bowel constipation over the years can back up poisons into the venous, arterial, and lymphatic systems and enter every cell of the body. Old fecal matter will balloon the bowel and weaken it, allowing bacterial toxins to enter the blood stream. The toxins then poison the nerves surrounding the colon, ultimately affecting all other related tissues, organs and systems.

Autointoxication is the result of constipation and a process whereby the body poisons itself by harboring a cesspool of decaying matter in the colon. It contains a high concentration of harmful bacteria. The toxins released by the decaying food gets into the bloodstream and goes to all parts of the body and weakens the entire system.

The ileocecal valve can become incompetent and cause regurgitation into the small intestine, which contains dangerous poisons to be reabsorbed into the blood stream. The incompetency of this valve is believed to be due to the enlargement of the cecum pulling the valve apart and preventing its closure.

The endocrine glands cannot handle the toxic load when the colon is backed up, and it becomes congested and unable to perform hundreds of functions vital to the health of the body. People who are constipated, and don't eliminate after every meal, could have several days or weeks of waste matter in their colon.

Natural Therapy: Lower bowel cleansing and blood purification is necessary. Colonics may be necessary to loosen the encrusted colon. Drink plenty of fresh fruit and vegetable juices. Exercise is essential for a healthy colon. Food combining and chewing food properly are vital to prevent constipation. Eat high-fiber foods.

Do sit-ups to reduce poor muscle tone which is usually present when constipation exists, causing pockets to form in the intestines that hold partially digested food. Practice deep breathing as oxygen is essential for respiration of all cells to detoxify waste material. Lack of oxygen can cause free radical formation and premature aging.

The colon is the principal organ for the detoxification of the lymph glands. Rebound exercises helps remove toxins from the lymph glands. Skin brushing promotes elimination.

Foods to Heal: Fresh lemon juice in water first thing in the morning will help. Include molasses, yogurt, wheat germ and bran in your diet. Soaked prunes, figs and raisins are healing as are raw beet, carrot and celery juices. Eat a lot of apples, peaches, berries, oranges, sprouted seeds, grains and nuts. Eat whole grains like millet, whole wheat, barley, buckwheat, oats, corn meal. Raw vegetable salads are an excellent way to add nutrition and bulk. Beans and lentils are are also excellent healing foods. Almond and sesame seed milk drinks lubricate the bowels.

Vitamins and Minerals: A steady supply of vitamin A is necessary to strengthen and repair the tissues. Vitamin C and bioflavonoids help control the sievability of cells. Supplement with vitamins B-complex, D, E (too much fat can cause deficiency of vitamin E), and K. Take a liquid multimineral, calcium and magnesium, selenium, zinc, and silicon. An iron deficiency may be related to toxins and poor elimination.

Herbal Combinations: Blood purifier, digestion, immune, liver and gallbladder, lower bowel, and red clover blends.

Single Herbs: Herbs have the ability to loosen hard material from the colon. Use aloe vera, alfalfa, barberry, buckthorn, burdock, cascara sagrada (cleans and rebuilds colon), comfrey, dandelion, fennel, fenugreek (loosens hard mucus), ginger, goldenseal, kelp, licorice, mullein, myrrh, pau d'arco, and psyllium. Psyllium is excellent for removing loosened material because it swells when taken with water, forming a bulky residue. It has the ability to absorb large quantities of sticky, gluey material along the colon walls. Senna (keeps colon clean), slippery elm (heals and nourishes colon) and yarrow are also beneficial.

Supplements: Apple pectin, acidophilus, chlorophyll, flaxseed, wheat grass, bentonite, fiber.

Avoid: Refined foods that cause constipation. Avoid laxatives—they are habit-forming and interfere with the proper absorption of sodium and potassium in the large intestine. Potassium is actually lost when laxatives are taken. Herbal laxatives, on the other hand, rebuild, heal and provide nutrients for a healthy colon. Dairy products are mucus-forming and constipating. Avoid mineral oil; it depletes vitamin A and other vitamins from the body. Avoid chemicals, additives and junk food which stress the body's ability to digest. Antibiotics destroy the bacterial flora in the colon.

✢ COUGHS

Coughing is a protective reflex, aimed at ridding the body of mucus, air pollution or irritants in the breathing apparatus. They vary in nature and severity. Some coughs are just a tickle in the throat that lasts for a few days and some are coughs that develop from a cold into bronchitis, pneumonia, asthma, tuberculosis or even cancer of the lungs. When a cough lasts more than a few weeks, care must be taken to look at the whole body and do some cleansing.

Poisons and toxins in the body make one susceptible to coughs, cold, flu and acute diseases. A low alkaline diet lowers resistance. Improper diet, as well as a lack of fresh air and exercise lowers vitality. Air pollution puts an extra burden on the lungs and lowers resistance to an already lowered system.

Different kinds of coughs are croupy, or hard, feverish, watery, catarrhal (phlegm), and chronic. Croupy cough usually comes on suddenly with a loud rasping sound. The phlegm is difficult to cough up, and it usually sounds worse than it really is. This cough is caused by inflammation of the larynx and trachea, with hardened and thick phlegm. A feverish cough comes on suddenly and is caused by an infection. If it is bronchitis the chest is tight and painful. A watery cough is usually caused from the nose draining down the throat. It is usually brought on during cold, wet weather when there is a lowered immune system. A catarrhal cough usually accompanies infections. It is worse when lying down. The cough produces thick, white phlegm, or thick white or green phlegm from the nose. It usually accompanies a cold. Chronic coughs are brought on because the initial cough was suppressed from eating with a cold or taking drugs for the cold. The mucus in the head area was never cleared out but was suppressed and hardened.

Natural Therapy: Change the diet to eliminate mucus from the stomach. The stomach and bowels need to be cleansed to keep the system in good working order. Stress can cause toxins to accumulate and put an extra burden on the immune system. A change of living habits is needed.

Foods to Heal: Citrus juices until the acute symptoms disappear. Vegetable broths, green drinks and herbal teas will help heal faster than eating food during acute disease.

Vitamins and Minerals: Vitamin A (high amounts at first), vitamin C with bioflavonoids (1,000 mg every hour at first), and B-complex (depleted fast during illness). Also take calcium, magnesium, potassium, selenium and zinc.

Herbal Combinations: Colds and flu, infection, lower bowel, nerves, potassium, red cover blend.

Single Herbs: Key herbs are alfalfa (tea), aloe vera (heals and prevents scar tissue), comfrey (healing), fenugreek (prevents mucus from forming and loosens hard mucus), garlic (kills germs and heal infections), ginger (settles stomach), goldenseal (kills germs, viruses and parasites), lobelia (removes obstructions), marshmallow, mullein, red raspberry, rose hips, slippery elm (for coughs and to heal throat and stomach). Other herbs are capsicum, dandelion, kelp, licorice, ma huang, passionflower (soothing for nerves), skullcap (feeds and heals nerves), and pau d'arco (cleans and kills germs).

Supplements: Green drinks, rice bran syrup, Chinese essential oils (external), peppermint tea, tea tree oil, and liquid herbal extracts.

Avoid: Stop eating during acute disease. The stomach needs to eliminate the mucus and toxins to repair and heal the body. Avoid antibiotics and drugs which only suppress the coughs and drainage.

✤ CROHN'S DISEASE

There are an ever-increasing number of people who are becoming afflicted with the disorder known as Crohn's disease. This is alarming

❖

because it is very serious. It is an inflammation of any portion of the GI tract, and extends through all layers of the intestinal wall.

The disease is characterized by scarring and narrowing of the colon, due to inflammation, and sometimes it is so severe that the colon becomes blocked and nothing can pass through. There is a lot of pain associated with this disease, which is often first manifested by diarrhea, weight loss, low stress tolerance, abdominal infections and anemia.

It is felt that Crohn's disease is an "autoimmune" disorder. It may be that the entire body (especially the gastrointestinal tract) becomes so toxic from many years of toxin buildup from medications, poor eating habits, etc., that the immune system becomes confused. It then attacks the toxic tissues, and begins to destroy them, thinking they are a foreign organism.

Many nutritionists feel that there is extreme parasite infestation associated with this disease. This further debilitates the immune system, of which Crohn's disease victims are already weak. An overburdened lymphatic system is another cause. High stress seems to be a factor. Young people (twelve years of age) are coming down with it. This indicates that maybe the mother's prenatal diet and postnatal diet for the child could be a factor.

Natural Therapy: A nutritional approach would be to cleanse, eliminate parasites, work with digestion and build the immune system. Blood purification and colon healing therapies. Drink plenty of liquids, pure water, herbal teas, fresh juices, wheat grass juice is healing. Watch food combining. Juice fasts are very healing. Add other foods after healing of the colon takes place.

Foods to Heal: Blend fresh and steamed vegetables and chew well foods such as broccoli, brussels sprouts, carrots, celery, cabbage, kale, and spinach. Herbs are very healing and provide vitamins and minerals and are considered food. Slippery elm is a food and will heal the colon. Use thermos cooking for delicious mush. Pour boiling water over whole grains, and let stand over night. Millet is easy to digest. Vegetable broths are healing and rich in minerals.

Vitamins and Minerals: Vitamins A and C are healing for the immune system. Bioflavonoids are necessary with the vitamin C. B-complex

❖

vitamins are necessary for proper digestion. B-vitamin deficiencies and poor absorption of nutrients are the major nutritional problems. Vitamins E along with A and C, help control infections. Multivitamin and mineral supplements are essential; deficiency is common in Crohn's disease. Selenium and zinc are also very healing. Vitamin K supplement is necessary.

Herbal Combinations: Anemia, glands, digestion, immune, potassium, lower bowel, ulcer.

Single Herbs: Aloe vera (healing), alfalfa (provides all minerals), dandelion, garlic, hops, kelp, lobelia, marshmallow, myrrh, papaya, pau d'arco, psyllium (healing and cleansing for the colon), saffron (helps in the assimilation of oils), skullcap (repairs nerves), slippery elm (food for the colon) and yellow dock.

Supplements: Essential fatty acids such as salmon oil, evening primrose oil, digestive enzymes, acidophilus (provides friendly bacteria in colon), liquid chlorophyll, glucomannan, flaxseed drink.

Avoid: Meat is hard on the digestive system, especially beef and pork. Sugar and all sugar products deplete essential nutrients. Avoid soft drinks, chocolate, candy cookies, cakes, all pastry products. Avoid caffeine, drugs, and all products that lower the immune system.

❖ CYSTIC FIBROSIS

Cystic Fibrosis is a genetic disorder—a recessive genetic trait—which has to be carried by both parents in order to have an afflicted child. The chances of having an affected child with cystic fibrosis when both parents carry those recessive genes is 25 percent. Most people never realize that they are carriers of these recessive genetic traits until they have a child with cystic fibrosis. It is the most common fatal genetic disease of Caucasian children.

Cystic fibrosis is a generalized dysfunction of the exocrine and endocrine systems in varying degrees of severity. The gastrointestinal effects of cystic fibrosis occur mainly in the intestines, pancreas and liver. One of the earliest such symptoms is 'meconium ileus'. The newborn with cystic fibrosis doesn't excrete meconium, a dark green mucilaginous material found in the intestine at birth. He develops symptoms of intestinal obstruction, such as abdominal distention, vomiting, constipation, dehydration and electrolyte imbalance. Eventually, obstruction of the pancreatic ducts and resulting deficiency of trypsin, amylase, and lipase prevent the conversion and absorption of fat and protein in the intestinal tract.

The undigested food is then excreted in frequent, bulky, foul smelling, pale stools with a high-fat content. The inability of the body to absorb nutrients produces poor weight gain, a ravenous appetite, sallow skin and distended abdomen. The inability to absorb fats produces deficiencies of the fat-soluble vitamins (A, E, and K), leading to clotting problems and retarded bone growth.

Natural Therapy: Blood purification and colon cleansing are essential. Carrot juice mixed with celery, cucumber, then beet juice, all in small amounts with larger amounts of carrot juice. Diet is very important.

Foods to Heal: Carrot juice with smaller amounts of beet, celery, cucumber. Wheat grass juice is healing and supplies protein and minerals and vitamins. Slippery elm added to juices will heal and also supply protein. Other mild foods can be added as strength is gained and healing is improved. Raw foods are essential to supply nutrients.

Vitamins and Minerals: Take beta-carotene to protect the mucous membranes and to prevent infections. Vitamin A derived from carrot juice will also supply calcium. Vitamin E is needed and vitamin C is essential to those with cystic fibrosis because they are plagued with frequent infections. Small frequent doses work better. All minerals are essential; they are easily lost with diarrhea.

Herbal Combinations: Anemia, glands, digestion, immune, lung, lower bowel.

Single Herbs: Key herbs are comfrey (healing), fennel (for digestion), ginger, lady's slipper (works on the medulla in the brain helping to regulate breathing, sweating, saliva and heart function), lobelia, marshmallow, mullein, papaya, peppermint, saffron (digests fats), and slippery elm. Other helpful herbs are pau d'arco, red clover, skullcap, kelp, dulse, and other sea weeds.

Supplements: Acidophilus, free-form amino acids, pancreatic digestive enzymes, chlorophyll, glucomannan (keeps colon clean), salmon oil, evening primrose oil, blue-green algae.

Avoid: Processed food, meat, too much cooked food, mucus-forming foods. Because of defects in the organs a thick, clogging mucus draws infections and obstructs the lungs and intestines. Avoid drugs, antibiotics, aspirin.

✤ CYSTS AND TUMORS

A cyst is a closed sac or pouch with a definite wall which contains fluid, semifluid or solid material. Tumors are a swelling or abnormal growth of tissues having no useful function in the body. Cancer cells are abnormal cells that invade healthy tissues. They travel through the system, and deposit themselves in the weakest areas of the body causing growths or tumors. Suppressing acute diseases can be the cause of cysts and tumors. Mucus is allowed to accumulate and harden in the body when acute diseases are not allowed to go through the five stages of healing.

Natural Therapy: Cleansing the blood and cells with short fasts, juices, and herbs to help loosen and eliminate the cysts and tumors.

Foods to Heal: High-fiber foods, deep yellow and dark green vegetables and fruits. Sweet potatoes, yams, squash, carrots, peaches, apricots.

Vitamins and Minerals: Vitamin A (destroys free radicals), B-complex (repairs cells), and vitamin C (heals and protects against cancer). Calcium, magnesium and potassium, selenium and zinc (protects the immune system).

Herbal Combinations: Blood purifier, digestion, immune, lower bowels, nerves.

Single Herbs: Burdock, chaparral (cleans and dissolves cysts and tumors), dandelion (cleans the liver), echinacea (cleans the lymphatics), garlic (kills germs), goldenseal (kills and destroys germ and acts as an antibiotic), kelp (healing and cleansing), milk thistle (helps heal liver), parsley, pau d'arco (purifies the blood), prickly ash (aids in circulation), red clover (red clover blend tea), suma (strengthens the body), yellow dock.

Supplements: Acidophilus, lecithin, liquid chlorophyll, salmon oil, wheat grass juice, fish oil lipids.

Avoid: Meat, white sugar, white flour products and fried foods. Eliminate antibiotics as they weaken the immune system, and stay

❖

away from caffeine, alcohol, chocolate, candy, cookies, pastries, all soft drinks. Avoid all food additives, and food colorings. Watch for sulfites and sulfates. Avoid smoking and using over-the-counter drugs.

❖ DEPRESSION

Depression is as common and widespread as the common cold or mental illness. Depression is a real affliction—it is not a sign of weakness. Neither is depression a hopeless condition. It can be treated nutritionally with successful results. The brain needs nutrition as much or more than the other organs of the body. The brain's neurotransmitters, which are responsible in regulating our behavior are controlled by the diet we eat.

Depression was called melancholia in the past. Many doctors found that autointoxication was the main cause of depression and mental problems. The brain is very sensitive to toxins. When the bowels are not kept clean, the toxins enter the blood and travel to the brain. One medical doctor wrote in an article in the *Medical Record* in 1937, "No matter how many stools or what their physical character may be..., marked retention of toxic or sapremic substances may exist. Many of the most toxic individuals that I have seen have daily and often more frequent bowel movements."

The World Health Organization conducted a survey and found that 200 million individuals worldwide suffer from depression. All of us face depression at one time or another in one form or another. Stressful situations cause depression. Normal depression comes with grief as in a death, divorce, loss of job, medical problems or other stressful situations. A mild chronic depression, where the "blues" continue, can be caused by negative feelings and a dissatisfaction with life. One loses interest in life, family and friends, and is often fatigued. There are also feelings of anger, anxiety and worthlessness.

Major depression can happen when one feels there is no relief in sight. There is usually change in sleeping habits. There is loss of appetite or some suffer from eating too much. The person may feel guilt and wish they were dead. They have feelings of anxiety, dread, worthlessness, and ill fate. This can also alternate with periods of normal behavior.

Manic depression is manifested by periods of high elation, working sprees, wild spending sprees, constant moving and action followed by deep depression.

Prozac is a popular, widely prescribed drug that doctors are using on three million people across the country for depression. It was approved by the FDA in December 1987 and was reported as having few side effects. This is a drug to be used carefully. The manufacturer admits that Prozac can cause agitation, hostility psychosis, and other frightening side effects such as "akathidia." Information of warning about Prozac states the following possible adverse nervous system reactions: abnormal dreams and agitation; infrequent abnormal gait, acute brain syndrome, akathisia, amnesia, apathy, delusions, depersonalization, euphoria, hallucinations, hostility, manic reaction, paranoid reaction, psychosis and vertigo. Rare side effects are abnormal electroencephalogram, antisocial reaction, chronic brain syndrome, and hysteria.

Natural Therapy: Blood and colon cleansing are necessary because toxins from the colon can enter the bloodstream and travel to the brain. Build the nervous system with herbs, fresh food and supplements. The circulatory system needs to be kept clean to supply oxygen and nutrients to the brain.

Foods to Heal: Complex carbohydrates such as brown rice, millet, buckwheat, corn meal, wheat, oats are good because they contain tryptophan, an amino acid that has a calming effect. Organically grown turkey breast is high in tryptophan. Protein creates alertness because it contains dopamine and norepinephrine. Fish is high in protein; salmon, cod, and tuna are good. Beans (dry) are high in protein. Fresh and steamed vegetables are rich in minerals which are essential for the brain and nervous system.

Vitamins and Minerals: Vitamin A, B-complex (with extra B$_6$, B$_{12}$, folic acid, niacin). Vitamin C and bioflavonoids along with B$_6$ are converted into brain neurotransmitters. Multiminerals are essential for brain health. Take extra calcium, magnesium, selenium and zinc.

Herbal Combinations: Blood purifier, bone, digestion, immune, lower bowels, potassium, nerve and stress combinations.

Single Herbs: Key herbs are gotu kola (brain food), capsicum (blood circulation), ginseng (energy food), kelp (cleans glands and veins), dong quai (tranquilizing on nerves), garlic (cleansing), chamomile (rich in calcium to feed the nerves). Herbs for the nerves are skullcap (rebuilds the nerves), hops (has sedative properties), passionflower (soothing on the nerves). Ginkgo (stimulates brain function) and suma (increases oxygen supply to the brain) are good for the brain. Other beneficial herbs are alfalfa, black cohosh, black walnut, burdock, chaparral, dandelion, ephedra, echinacea, ginger, goldenseal, hawthorn, ho-shou-wu, lady's slipper, licorice, lobelia, red raspberry, red clover, wood betony, and yellow dock.

Supplements: Bee pollen, spirulina, chlorophyll, essential fatty acids such as evening primrose oil, salmon oil, blue-green algae, lecithin.

Avoid: Heavy metal poisoning. Severe depression can be a symptom of lead poisoning, or other metals. Allergies can also cause severe depression. Caffeine addiction creates thiamine deficiency and weakens the nervous system, and the lack of other B-vitamins can cause depression. Avoid junk food as it puts a double stress on the body and dulls the appetite for wholesome food. Sugar throws the body out of balance, harms the pancreas and depletes essential B-vitamins and calcium from the body. Too much meat causes uric acid and other toxins to accumulate in the blood. Alcohol creates a lot of hard work for the detoxifying organs (the liver, kidneys, pancreas), and also depletes vitamins and minerals. Constant stress will cause the nerves to weaken and put a burden on the glands and organs of the body. Learn stress management through relaxation, meditation, and exercise.

❖ DIABETES

More than ten million Americans have diabetes and the number is growing. It is estimated that two out of five people with diabetes do not realize they have the disease. People with diabetes are up to four times more likely to die from a heart attack, and people with diabetes have a greater risk of having strokes. Symptoms are excessive thirst and urination, and excessive hunger. General weakness and depression, skin disorders, including boils and vaginal infections, blurred vision, tingling leg cramps, impotence, and a dry mouth are other frequent complaints.

There are two types of diabetes. The first is Type 1 or juvenile diabetes mellitus, also called insulin dependent diabetes mellitus (IDDM).

❖

In this type of diabetes the pancreas does not produce insulin, the hormone that is responsible for moving the sugar in the blood into the cells. This is a more serious diabetes and almost always develops in childhood.

In Type 2 diabetes the pancreas is producing insulin, but the cells have too few chemical receptors and the cells starve, resulting in lack of energy The major cause of Type 2 is thought to be obesity. Overeating and eating the wrong kinds of food are the major cause. It is like you are starving your body while eating a lot of food.

Natural Therapy: Blood purification, bowel cleansing through enemas, colonics or lower bowel cleansers. A change of diet is required. Fasting will help eliminate sugar from the cells in the body. Short fasts are very important to prevent weakening the body before it is strong enough to handle long fasts. Exercise and skin brushing will speed the cleansing and healing of the body. Exercise helps the body use up excess blood sugar. Thirty to sixty minutes of aerobic exercise a day benefits the body for up to twelve hours. A diet change is the biggest challenge a diabetic has. It is sometimes hard to change eating habits.

Foods to Heal: Sprouted grains added to salads and vegetable casseroles are recommended, as are non-starchy vegetables, lightly steamed. Excellent vegetables are asparagus, green beans, okra, celery, watercress, parsley alfalfa, and Jerusalem artichokes (a starch the pancreas can handle). Goat milk and whey powder are high in sodium. Eat sprouts (alfalfa, bean, radish and fenugreek), garlic, onions endive, fresh fruits and berries, beets, and leafy green vegetables. A high-fiber diet helps to lower blood triglycerides in diabetics and pre-diabetics. Fiber also has the ability to repair faulty sugar metabolism by its complex effect on stomach and intestinal functioning. Psyllium hulls and grains such whole oats, wheat, millet, buckwheat, barley, and brown rice should be included in the diet.

Vitamins and Minerals: Natural vitamin A is the best as beta-carotene is difficult for a diabetic to convert into vitamin A. All vitamins are involved directly or indirectly in maintaining normal sugar metabolism. B-complex vitamins help to cut down on insulin intake, and strengthen and repair nerves. Vitamin C with bioflavonoids is essential for artery health, cleans the veins and strengthens the immune system. Vitamin E is necessary to help the body store sugar as glycogen. It also helps iron to be absorbed by the thyroid, cutting down on artery complications. Amino acids are also important: L-carnitine and L-glutamine help the liver to metabolize fat.

All minerals are essential for the diabetic. Chromium helps the body to stabilize blood sugar. Copper aids the body in utilizing enzymes and protein assimilation. Calcium is vital for the nerves when used along with magnesium to balance the body. Biotin and inositol, found in lecithin, are essential for all body functions. Silicon is essential for cleaning the body to improve the health of diabetics. Zinc is one of the main ingredients of insulin and a lack of zinc is seen in diabetics. Potassium is also necessary for diabetics.

Herbal Combinations: Blood purifier, bone, lower bowels, pancreas and diabetes, parasites and worms, potassium and stress.

Single Herbs: Key herbs are alfalfa, aloe vera, black walnut (kills parasites), buchu, burdock (cleans blood), cedar berries (heals the pancreas), cornsilk, dandelion, garlic, gentian, goldenseal (acts as insulin, stops internal bleeding), hawthorn, horsetail, kelp and psyllium. Other beneficial herbs are capsicum, chaparral, echinacea, ginger, ginseng, Irish moss, juniper berries, licorice, lobelia, myrrh, parsley, queen of the meadow, red clover, uva ursi, watercress, wormwood and yellow dock.

Supplements: Liquid chlorophyll, blue-green algae, lecithin, glucomannan, rice bran syrup, salmon oil, evening primrose oil, and digestive enzymes.

Avoid: Heavy meat diet, soft drinks, caffeine, tobacco, heavy starches, and all denatured foods. Avoid all sugar products—they are the downfall of the diabetic—as well as white flour products. Food containing refined carbohydrates causes the blood sugar to rise quite high during the first two or three hours after eating (diabetes) but then it plunges very low in the fourth hour, giving symptoms of low blood sugar (hypoglycemia). This soon wears out the pancreas because it has to constantly produce excessive insulin.

❖ DIARRHEA AND DYSENTERY

Diarrhea and dysentery are the ways nature takes care of cleansing the body quickly of distress. They can be caused from toxic bacteria, colitis,

❖

parasites, viruses, chemicals, allergies, antibiotics (destroy friendly bacteria) or food poisoning. Diarrhea can be acute or chronic and the condition can be dangerous, especially for babies and young children, because it can lead to a loss of body fluids and salts. When a child becomes weak with sunken eyes a doctor should be contacted.

Diarrhea is usually the result of unfriendly bacteria invading the intestinal tract. Poorly cleaned dishes, glasses and silverware can also cause diarrhea. A cutting board can become contaminated if you cut raw meat or chop vegetables or fruit without using a disinfectant. Some forms of bacteria cause throwing up which helps eliminate contaminated food from the stomach. When contaminated food passes on to the intestinal tract, it causes diarrhea. If it enters the blood stream, it will cause an infection and if the immune system is low, fevers, headaches and other discomforts will occur.

Natural Therapy: Cleansing the digestive system through fasting is the best way to heal and improve diarrhea and dysentery. Enemas will also speed up healing. Catnip tea is mild and healing for children. It can be used as an enema as well as taken internally. Slippery elm supplies nutrients and speeds recovery from diarrhea. Use pure water and vegetable juices, especially carrot juice. Rice water and barley water will heal the digestive system.

Foods to Heal: Bananas contain pectin which will tighten up loose bowels. Carob normalizes the bowels. Unsweetened yogurt is also good.

Vitamins and Minerals: Vitamins A and C will heal the digestive system. B-complex vitamins are lost during diarrhea so supplement. Vitamin E is needed for calcium assimilation and to protect the cells and veins. Multiminerals are necessary as they are lost during diarrhea. Take extra calcium, potassium, and zinc.

Herbal Combinations: Blood purifier, colitis, congestion, lower bowels, nerves, and potassium.

Single Herbs: Slippery elm is the best herb for diarrhea and dysentery; it will help heal and regulate. Goldenseal is also a great healer of the digestive system, and it kills parasites that can cause diarrhea. Other key herbs are capsicum (kills germs), comfrey (soothes and heals irritated mucous membranes), chamomile tea (soothing on nerves), gar-

❖

lic (kills bacteria, parasites and worms), gentian (heals the digestive system), ginger (stops cramps), kelp (replaces minerals lost in diarrhea), pau d'arco (kills bacteria), raspberry tea (heals and soothes), and white oak bark (heals). Other herbs to help are alfalfa, bayberry, dandelion, hawthorn, licorice, lobelia, myrrh, oatstraw (supplies minerals), red clover, and wormwood.

Supplements: Acidophilus (replaces bacteria lost in diarrhea), charcoal tablets (absorb toxins and gases), blackberry juice (unsweetened), chlorophyll, glucomannan, and evening primrose oil. Carob powder is handy to have in controlling diarrhea.

Avoid: Stop eating heavy foods in order to give the digestive system a rest and help the body heal itself. Avoid sugar products as they irritate the digestive system. Antibiotics destroy friendly bacteria.

❖ Diverticulitis

Diverticula are small, pouch-like areas in the large colon. The condition known as diverticulitis occurs when food enters the pockets of the large colon and causes infections and toxins to accumulate. Constipation and a low-fiber diet are the main cause of this problem. Straining from hard stools causes pockets in the colon to form, allowing toxins to accumulate. Diverticulitis is another form of autointoxication. Symptoms are similar to appendicitis except on the left-hand side. There is tenderness, cramping and fever. Chronic diverticulitis can cause irregular bowels, constipation and some pain.

Diverticulitis is very common, striking nearly 70 percent of people over the age of seventy. It usually begins with persistent constipation, which can alternate with diarrhea. It can cause nausea, vomiting, abdominal swelling, cramps and pain. It can even bring a flu-like feeling of chills and fever. Complications may develop, causing problems in the bladder, small intestine and uterus. Hemorrhaging and rectal bleeding can occur.

Natural Therapy: The average medical doctor will usually prescribe a low-residue, soft diet for people with diverticulitis. But today it is pretty well established that this diet is what created the disease in the first place. A high-fiber diet from whole grains, fruit and vegetables is essential. The first therapy is to use demulcent herbs to speed the heal-ing. It is also beneficial to use lower bowel therapy to clean and build up the lower bowels. Blood purifiers are necessary to clean the organs.

Foods to Heal: Cooked grains such as millet, buckwheat, oats (whole), wheat, yellow corn meal, and barley. They should be cooked in a ther-mos overnight to retain all the enzymes for digestion. Wheat grass juice speeds healing as do carrot, celery and beet juice. Steamed veg-etables should be blended for easy digestion and assimilation until healing takes place.

Vitamins and Minerals: Vitamin A heals and protects the mucus mem-branes and vitamin C heals and protects immune system. Vitamin B-complex improves the tone of intestinal tract and builds the blood. A vitamin K deficiency can cause intestinal disorders. All minerals are needed (liquid are better for easy assimilation). Take extra calcium, magnesium, chromium, silicon and zinc.

Herbal Combinations: Bone (rich in minerals), comfrey and pepsin (comfrey heals and pepsin dissolves toxins), colitis, digestion, lower bowels, ulcers.

Single Herbs: Key herbs are aloe vera (heals), alfalfa (rich in minerals as well as vitamin K), comfrey, fenugreek (cleans and heals colon), gar-lic (an antibiotic), glucomannan (cleans colon), hops (relaxing to colon), kelp (provides minerals), marshmallow (healing), papaya, psyllium (food for the colon), slippery elm (soothes and heals colon), and red clover tea. Other beneficial herbs are dandelion, lobelia, myrrh, pau d'arco, skullcap, and yellow dock.

Supplements: Acidophilus (milk-free), liquid chlorophyll, aloe vera juice, bentonite, fish oil lipids, salmon oil, fiber supplements, high-fiber cookies.

Avoid: Meat (hard to digest), dairy products and low-fiber foods. Eliminate all white sugar and flour products—they lack fiber and nourishment.

✢ Ear Problems (Otitis media)

Ear infections are a common childhood complaint. Autointoxication is the cause of most ear infections. The blood is poisoned through absorption of toxic material from the intestinal canal. A child may be born with a weakened system, or can acquire toxins with a diet of milk products. Another cause may be feeding baby cereal to a child before the body produces the enzyme needed for the digestion of grains. Bacteria then develops in the ears as a result of the accumulation of toxins.

A huge number of antibiotics are prescribed each year for ear infections but cases of children with chronic middle ear diseases have only increased since the advent of antibiotics. Antibiotics can cause fluid retention in the ear and prevent healing. A blockage of the eustachian tube is the most common cause of infection. Mucus or inflammation is produced when a cold develops, when respiratory infections are present, or when a child suffers from allergies or childhood diseases such as measles, chickenpox, and strep throat. Together the mucus and inflammation can block a child's eustachian tube, which is shorter than an adult's and can get plugged easily.

Be aware that foreign objects in the ear and nose are also common causes of earaches. I worked for an ear, eyes and nose specialist, and many children were brought in for removal of beans, pieces of paper, cotton balls, jelly beans, pieces of cereal and even safety pins or paper clips. Such objects may cause pain or lead to infections. Parents become concerned because of the pain children suffer. The pain is usually caused by pressure that develops when infections interfere with the drainage of the ear through the eustachian tubes. But, according to Dr. Robert Mendelsohn, hearing loss from ear infections is very rare.

Natural Therapy: Blood purification, enemas or lower bowel cleansing will speed the healing. A cleansing diet using citrus juices with liquid or powdered vitamin C will heal and clean up infections. Mullein oil in the ears will help with the pain and garlic and olive oil will heal infection. Lobelia drops also help to ease the pain. If the eardrum is broken, don't put anything in the ear until a doctor has cleaned it out. Applying a warm towel soaked in catnip or chamomile tea will ease the pain. You can alternate the warm towel with a cold towel (not ice) to stimulate circulation and speed healing. Soak the feet in hot water with added tablespoon of mustard or ginger. Roast a lemon in the oven and put a few drops of the juice in the ear (very healing). Earaches usually clear up within three to five days by themselves.

❖

Foods to Heal: Freshly juiced citrus fruits, tree-ripened if possible, and carrot juice (high in vitamins A and calcium) are excellent. Vegetable juices and vegetable broths made with celery, potato skins, parsley, and any root and green leafy vegetables should be given to the child.

Vitamins and Minerals: Vitamin A, E or cod liver oil for children help control infections. Vitamin C along with calcium helps in healing and preventing infections. B-complex vitamins are healing. Take a multimineral for healing, with extra silicon, selenium and zinc.

Herbal Combinations: Blood purifiers, lower bowel cleansers, bone combinations.

Single Herbs: Key herbs are echinacea (natural antibiotic), fenugreek (loosens mucus), garlic (natural antibiotic), ginger (settles stomach), goldenseal (heals), hops (relaxes), lobelia (cleans stomach), red clover (cleans blood), skullcap, valerian and yellow dock. Other beneficial herbs are aloe vera, bayberry, bilberry, black walnut, burdock, capsicum, chaparral, comfrey, gotu kola, grapevine, kelp, lady's slipper, oatstraw, passionflower and wood betony.

Supplements: Liquid chlorophyll, acidophilus, green drinks, lemon juice in warm water with pure maple syrup. Herbal teas such as chamomile, alfalfa-mint and red raspberry are beneficial. Essential fatty acids are very healing and essential for children as well as adults. Use salmon oil, evening primrose oil or grind flaxseed to a fine powder and mix with juice or water.

Avoid: Milk products. They are mucus-forming and increase toxin accumulation. Avoid sugar and white flour products. Avoid a heavy meat diet; use more grains, beans, seeds and nut milk.

❖ ENDOMETRIOSIS

Endometriosis is a rather common disease in our present age. It is estimated that 40 to 60 percent of women who undergo hysterectomies have endometriosis. It is an outgrowth of the uterine lining into the pelvic cavity that can cause irregular bleeding, pain during intercourse and/or menstruation, severe pelvic pain and even infertility.

This condition was discovered in 1899 and described in medical journals. In 1920 Dr. I. A. Sampson described the ever increasing disease as very serious. Sampson found clumps of brown, sticky tissue and

❖

old, clotted blood adhering in unusual places: ovaries, rectal ligaments, intestines, and fallopian tubes, causing infertility to increase at a very high rate. In severe cases, the abdominal organs were glued together and twisted out of place by the contortions of the unusual tissue. Then he discovered that the sticky, clotted tissue was the same as that which lined the normal uterus. It also reacted to the hormonal cycle the same way as the uterine tissue, proliferating when stimulated by estrogen and actually bleeding during menstruation.

The reason endometriosis is hard to diagnosis is that it can appear and disappear according to the hormonal profile of the woman. It is not fully understood how the tissue escapes from the uterus in the first place. One theory is that the excess uterine lining is forced upward and out through the fallopian tubes by heavy menstrual contractions. Another theory is that endometrial tissue develops from simple, undifferentiated epithelial cells in the abdomen, like what essentially happens in the female fetus during early pregnancy. Today physicians realize that endometriosis can probably arise from both of these theories: retrograde menstruation and inappropriate epithelial cell proliferation. Some doctors feel that it also stems from other causes not yet recognized—episiotomies, IUDs, cauterization of the cervix and even laparoscopy.

The reason this disease is more prevalent is because of the excess estrogen in beef, chicken, turkey, and all dairy products: milk, butter, cottage cheese, sour cream, cream cheese and whipping cream. Excess toxins, such as artificial hormones, would be handled better by the body if we kept the colon healthy and regular. When excess toxins are present, the liver becomes overloaded because the bowels are backed up. As a result toxins enter the blood stream and cause problems in the areas where estrogen is used—the breasts, uterus, vagina and other related parts.

In 1984 an epidemic of early puberty was reported in both males and females all across Puerto Rico. Enlarged breasts in pre-teen children were also reported by health authorities in parts of the continental United States.

Dr. Saenz de Rodriguez of Puerto Rico had seen many cases of premature puberty for several years. She became convinced that children were being contaminated with estrogen, causing four and five-year-old

❖

girls to suffer from enlarged breasts and ovarian cysts. Milk products, beef and poultry were found to be the problem. She said "we are supposed to mind our manners and not question the effects that drugs have upon the population, or your colleagues call you a trouble-maker. Much of what we consider 'healthful growth' in our youngsters could be similar to the fattening process the ranchers now use for their cattle. We should not, however, ignore the time-bomb that is present in those sky-rocketing sales figures for fried food among young people."

Natural Therapy: Blood purification and lower bowel therapy will clean and purify the body of excess estrogen and other toxins. Change to a diet using fresh juices from vegetables and fruits. Fruits are cleansing and vegetables are builders with their high mineral content. Instead of a high-meat diet change to brown rice, grains, beans, lentils, peas, and all natural food. Exercise is very beneficial to prevent adhesions from adhering to the walls of the uterus and other organs. It also helps to normalize hormone levels by metabolizing fat. Any aerobic activity stimulates the release of endorphins which are natural opiates that produce a sense of well-being and protect against pain.

Foods to Heal: Vegetables, steamed and fresh, and fresh salads using leaf lettuce, cabbage, carrots, broccoli, and all vegetables. Use olive oil and lemon juice for dressing with garlic, onions, parsley, and vegetable seasonings. Use brown rice, millet, buckwheat, and all whole grains. Thermos cooking will retain the enzymes and B-complex vitamins. Be sure and drink the liquid used to thermos cook. It is rich in enzymes for digestion. Sunflower and sesame seeds and almonds and almond milk are also beneficial. When eliminating sugar, alcohol, caffeine drinks, chocolate and refined foods, and at the same time adding B-complex, some women may at first experience a worsening of symptoms. This is because the ovaries are responding to good nutrition and speed up estrogen production. But with a good diet and clean bowels the liver is able to eliminate the excess estrogen.

Vitamins and Minerals: Vitamins A and E help heal and protect against scar tissue, as well as aid in hormone imbalance. Vitamin C and bioflavonoids are essential in healing and cleansing the body. B-complex vitamins are very important. They are lost every day, and stress

❖

rapidly depletes the body of these vitamins. Extra B6 with magnesium will reduce symptoms of estrogen overload. Remember the liver is the site of eliminating excess estrogen, and it cannot do it without adequate B vitamins. Multiminerals are very important, especially iron (found in yellow dock), iodine (found in kelp), and calcium and magnesium found in calcium herbal formulas. Selenium, zinc and silicon are also necessary.

Herbal Combinations: Blood purifiers, female glands, immune, lower bowels, nerves, and stress.

Single Herbs: Key herbs are black cohosh, cramp bark, damiana, dong quai, false unicorn, gentian, ginseng, gotu kola, kelp, licorice, sarsaparilla, saw palmetto, squaw vine and wild yam. Other important herbs are alfalfa, black walnut, burdock (cleans blood), capsicum (circulation to speed healing), chapparal (cleans blood and liver), dandelion (cleans liver), garlic, ginger, goldenseal (clears infections), ho-shou-wu, hawthorn, Irish moss, lobelia, mistletoe, myrrh, red clover (blood cleanser), skullcap (cleans veins and restores nerves), watercress, wood betony, wormwood and yellow dock.

Supplements: Free-form amino acids, essential fatty acids in salmon and fish liver oils, lecithin, spirulina, pancreatic enzymes, and hydrochloric acid if needed. Chlorophyll cleans the blood.

Avoid: All products that have hormones added: meat, poultry, milk, cheese, cottage cheese, butter, sour cream, whipping cream. Avoid sugar, it depletes the body of necessary B-complex vitamins and calcium. Avoid estrogen therapies, if possible. Caffeine and chocolate also aggravate female problems.

❖ ENVIRONMENTAL POISONING

Environmental toxins are a real health problem. They are in our water, food and air. Herbicide and pesticide residues are everywhere. We are constantly being exposed, and residue samples are found in the blood and urine of people living in both urban and rural areas. They have also been found in mothers' milk. These poisons are capable of causing mutations and cancer.

Lindane (bug bombs) are used in home gardens and on farms for treating seeds and hardwood lumber. Insecticides are also found in animal shampoos, flea collars, shelf paper and floor wax. They can cause cancer, are toxic to a growing fetus, damage the reproductive organs and children are very susceptible.

We are also threatened with electromagnetic radiation, which has been linked to leukemia. We have food additives, preservatives, artificial coloring, sprays on our fruits to ripen them artificially, and colors to enhance their selling ability. We are bombarded with all kinds of pollution. Radiation poisoning suppresses an already weakened immune system. When you undergo radiation therapy you may experience radiation burns, scarring, fatigue and a strain on the immune system. Radiation destroys many nutrients in the body. Supplements are vital to improve immune function and protect the system of diseases.

Natural Therapy: Keep the immune system strong and the liver clean in order to eliminate the toxins we breathe and eat. Blood, liver and lower bowels need to be kept clean and in good working order. We need to demand food that is free from additives and other chemicals.

Foods to Heal: Green leafy vegetables, whole grains, beans, high-fiber foods, broccoli, cabbage, kale, carrots, spinach, green peppers.

Vitamins and Minerals: Vitamin A helps detoxify toxins as well as protect the immune system; B-complex protects the cells with extra B_5, B_6, and B_{12} to protect against stress; vitamin C with bioflavonoids heals and protects the immune system; and vitamin E protects against free radicals, and heals and protects against radiation burns. Minerals are essential. They act as chelating agents to metals and other toxins. Calcium helps take lead out of the body and selenium and zinc protect the immune system. Silicon helps protect the bones.

Herbal Combinations: Blood purifiers, chelating, bone (rich in minerals), immune formulas, nerve and stress formulas. Lower bowel formulas help to eliminate toxins the liver filters.

Single Herbs: Alfalfa, aloe vera (heals and protects against burns), burdock (purifies blood and eliminates toxins), capsicum (increases circulation for rapid healing), chaparral (cleans blood and eliminates poisons), comfrey (healing), echinacea (cleans blood and lymphatic system), garlic (natural antibiotic), ginkgo (healing and promotes brain function), goldenseal (healing for mucous membranes), juniper

❖

berries, kelp (supplies minerals to eliminate poisons), lobelia, mullein, parsley, pau d'arco (cleans blood and protects liver), red clover (blood cleanser), sarsaparilla, suma, watercress and yellow dock.

Supplements: Acidophilus, liquid chlorophyll, bee pollen, blue-green algae, wheat grass juice, barley green drinks, germanium, coenzyme Q$_{10}$, amino acids (L-carnitine, glutathione, L-methionine, L-cysteine).

Avoid: Avoid all food additives. Frozen food contains a lot of preservatives. Don't smoke. Second-hand tobacco smoke will harm the lungs and children are very susceptible to smoke. Avoid sugar and all white flour products. Meat has antibiotics and hormones and fried foods will weaken the immune system.

❖ EPILEPSY

In his book *The Ultimate Healing System,* Donald LePore, N.D., states, "We believe that epilepsy is not a disease, but is actually nature's way of getting rid of the deteriorating matter on the brain. The epileptic seizure is like an electrical storm; this is nature's way of giving an electrical charge to correct the malfunction of the brain which sometimes is scar tissue in the area."

The actual epileptic seizure is due to a sudden, abnormal and excessive electrical discharge within the brain. In primary epilepsy the basic cause is unknown, but there is usually a genetic predisposition. Secondary epilepsy can be from a head injury, bacterial meningitis or malaria. It is often associated with cerebral palsy, mental retardation, brain tumors and cysts and hydrocephalus.

There are also drugs that can cause epilepsy or aggravate existing epileptic disorders: amphetamines, antihistamines, chloroquine, cimetidine, cycloserine, monoamine oxidase inhibitors, oral contraceptives, phenothiazines, tricyclic antidepressants. Dilantin is the most widely prescribed medication for epilepsy. It works on the motor cortex to stop the spread of seizure activity. There are, however, precautions when using this drug; it can cause mental confusion, dizziness, vomiting and constipation.

❖

Natural Therapy: Blood purification and lower bowel cleansing. Prevent toxins from entering the blood by keeping the bowels moving every day. A high-fiber diet with wholesome food will help nourish the brain and nervous system. The brain is very sensitive to toxins from the blood.

Foods to Heal: Fresh fruit and juices, raw and steamed vegetables, whole grains, sprouts from seeds and grains, green drinks, and raw food to nourish the brain and nerves. Thermos cooking of grains helps to retain enzymes, and vitamins and minerals essential for brain nourishment. Fresh green salads should be eaten every day.

Vitamins and Minerals: B-complex vitamins, especially folic acid and B_{12}, which are quickly destroyed when taking dilantin or phenobarbital. All B vitamins are important. Vitamins A, C and E provide protection to the immune system. Choline is needed to form acetylcholine, a major neurotransmitter that can improve memory. Minerals are essential for brain health. Sodium deficiency can cause brain malfunction. Calcium and magnesium feed and nourish the brain and nervous system. Selenium, silicon and zinc help to nourish the gland and brain. Manganese deficiency is seen in epileptics. B_6 helps to prevent convulsions.

Herbal Combinations: Blood cleanser, digestion, glands, nerve, lower bowels. Herbs are very beneficial to the nervous system and brain function.

Single Herbs: Key herbs are black walnut (parasites can cause epilepsy), burdock (cleans blood), capsicum, echinacea (cleans glands), garlic, ginkgo (stimulates brain), gotu kola (food for the brain), hawthorn, hops (nerves), lady's slipper (strengthens brain function), lobelia, passionflower, pau d'arco (cleans blood and liver), red clover, skullcap (brain relaxer), valerian. Other important herbs are alfalfa, black cohosh, dandelion, gentian, ginger, licorice and yellow dock.

Supplements: Acidophilus, lecithin, psyllium, glucomannan, bee pollen, spirulina, senna tea, rice bran syrup. Hydrochloric acid aids in digestion and the removal of toxic material that interferes with brain function. Taurine, tryptophan and glutamine detoxify ammonia from the brain. All amino acids are essential for brain health. Chlorophyll cleans the blood.

❖

Avoid: Avoid all denatured food. Sugar is detrimental to the body as well as the brain. White flour lacks essential minerals and fiber. Tobacco, caffeine and alcohol are very harmful to the brain and nervous system. Avoid fried foods as they cause free radicals and destruction to the cells.

❖ EPSTEIN-BARR VIRUS

Epstein-Barr virus is also called chronic fatigue syndrome and the "fatigue disease." It is becoming widespread and is a common virus that usually remains dormant in most people, but when the immune system is lowered can be triggered. It has been around for a long time and causes infectious mononucleosis. The Epstein-Barr virus causes both chronic fatigue and mono, but mononucleosis strikes all at once, hits hard and usually lasts two to four weeks. Chronic fatigue can linger for months and maybe even years.

Epstein-Barr virus symptoms are: fatigue that leaves you exhausted, recurrent upper-respiratory tract infections, swollen lymph nodes, memory loss, achy joints and muscles, low-grade fevers, headaches, night sweats, poor concentration, irritability, and serious depression. In the past, Epstein-Barr has been misdiagnosed as a psychosomatic problem. Truly, however, Epstein-Barr depletes the body's natural immunity and leaves a person susceptible to a number of illnesses.

Natural Therapy: Blood purification and lower bowel cleanse. Short fasts to clean the blood, using juices and pure water. Carrot, celery and parsley juices as well as green drinks purify the blood. Bed rest and relaxation therapy will help speed healing.

Foods to Heal: Citrus fruit (rich in vitamin C), cherries, parsley, green peppers, watercress, kale, broccoli, fresh salads with lots of raw vegetables.

Vitamins and Minerals: Vitamin A builds the immune system, as does B-complex. Vitamin C with bioflavonoids strengthens the immune system and heals. A multimineral is healing and essential for the body. Take extra selenium, silicon and zinc.

Herbal Combinations: Blood purifier (red clover blends), digestion, infection (containing herbs and vitamins), liver (helps to detoxify the toxins), nerve and stress herbal formulas.

❖

Single Herbs: Key herbs are echinacea (cleans glands), garlic (antibiotic), goldenseal (cleans and heals), horsetail, lobelia, oatstraw, pau d'arco (blood cleanser), red clover, saffron (helps to stop aches and pains), skullcap (helps the nerves). Other beneficial herbs are aloe vera, buchu, burdock, capsicum, comfrey, cornsilk, dandelion, ginger, hawthorn, licorice, myrrh, parsley, watercress and yellow dock.

Supplements: Bee pollen, acidophilus, evening primrose oil or salmon oil, garlic oil, chlorophyll and rice bran syrup.

Avoid: Sugar depletes calcium and B-vitamins. Caffeine drinks lower the immune system and deplete potassium and other minerals from the body. Avoid fried foods, high-fat foods, white sugar products and antibiotics—they will not help in viruses.

❖ Eye Problems

Eyesight is a precious gift. At least 80 percent of the decisions we make each day are based on information we receive with vision. Yet more than ten million people in the United States suffer severe vision disability and the medical profession gives them no hope. The drugs prescribed and the surgeries performed offer no relief.

Retinitis pigmentosa, an inherited genetic eye disease, occurs when the retina's nerve elements cause progressive atrophy, clumping of pigment and finally atrophy of the optic disks. Night blindness is one of the first signs. Other diseases of the eyes are senile macular degeneration, diabetic retinopathy, optic nerve atrophy and cataracts. All of these will increase blindness by 60 percent in the next forty years.

In the United States many eye specialists feel that clogged blood vessels are big contributors to blindness. The eye, along with the brain, requires more nutrition and circulation than any other single body organ. Poor nutrition clogs up tiny arteries, veins, and capillaries that support the visual system. The gradual clogging, which has been traced to poor nutrition, can result in eventual cataracts, blindness, and other visual problems.

Common drugs also have an adverse effect on the eyes. Sedative drugs such as tranquilizers and sleeping pills destroy the electrochemical balance, interfering with nerve transmission by putting out "foreign energies" as well as preventing vital nutrients from entering the eyes.

❖

Air pollution, especially tobacco smoke, can cause burning, dry, itchy, irritated and bloodshot eyes. Iridology can help determine weaknesses in other parts of the body. In fact, eye problems are often an early indication of diseases in the body. Dark circles under the eyes are a sign of allergies, watery and red eyes are a sign of a cold coming on, bulging eyes can indicate a thyroid problem. Yellowing of the eyes is an indication of hepatitis, liver problems or gallbladder problems. An eye specialist can see signs of high blood pressure and diabetes in patients when doing a regular eye examination.

Natural Therapy: Good nutrition is vital to maintain good eyesight and prevention is always better than the cure. Blood purification, and lower bowel cleansing are essential. A natural herbal eyewash will cleanse and stimulate circulation to the eye tissues. Use often to prevent the clogging of tiny capillaries and veins. The eyes absorb toxins from the lower bowel, part of a process known as autointoxication, or self poisoning. A liver cleanse and bowel cleanse with enemas, colonics or lower bowel cleansers will improve eyesight and other problems. It just takes patience and perseverance. Foot reflexology is another thing that has a direct stimulating effect on the eyes and brain. It will help promote circulation in the eye area.

Foods to Heal: Whole grain (thermos cooking to retain the enzymes), millet, buckwheat, whole oats, wheat, barley, and all whole grains, brown rice, yellow corn meal, beans of all kinds. Green leafy vegetables, whole nuts and seeds, and a lot of raw and steamed vegetables. Avocados are high in vitamin A and protein. Carrots and raw carrot juice are rich in vitamin A and calcium.

Vitamins and Minerals: Vitamin A helps prevent night blindness, protects the eyes from irritations, and protects from dry eyes. B-complex vitamins help prevent eye sensitivity and itching. A B_2 deficiency shows in people with itching, eye irritation, and poor adaptability to light changes. Niacin clears out the fatty deposits from tiny blood vessels, and improves blood flow. B_6 will lower ocular pressure and inositol is necessary for healthy eye membranes. Vitamin C with bioflavonoids is abundant in the lens of the eyes and protects against the formation of cataracts. Vitamins C and E protect against cellular deterioration caused by smoke, junk food and air pollution and both carry oxygen to the cells. Prolonged mineral deficiency can result in squinting, distorted visual perception, vertigo, fatigue, headaches and painful eyes. Zinc is necessary for the transformation of vitamin A. Chromium and zinc protect against cataracts. Calcium is important to the connective tissues of the eyes. Deficiency results in a softening of the outer shell of the eyeball.

Herbal Combinations: Blood purifiers, digestion, eye formulas, infection (when infected), lower bowels and stress.

Single Herbs: Key herbs are bilberry (strengthens eyes), capsicum (cleans capillaries), eyebright (improves eyes), goldenseal (cleans veins), hops, lobelia, passionflower (improves nerves), skullcap and valerian. Other beneficial herbs are aloe vera, bayberry, black cohosh, black walnut, burdock, chaparral, comfrey, echinacea, fenugreek, garlic, ginger, ginseng, gotu kola, grapevine, hawthorn, myrrh, oatstraw, red clover, white oak and yellow dock.

Supplements: Evening primrose oil, salmon oil, cod liver oil, chlorophyll and lecithin. Taurine, an amino acid, protects tissues under stress. Free-form amino acids are essential for eye health.

Avoid: Caffeine has an adverse effect on the ability of the eyes to focus for reading or other close work. Sugar depletes calcium and B-vitamins that are essential for eye health. Cigarette smoke is very harmful on the eyes. Tinted eyeglasses prevent light from entering the eyes.

❖ FATIGUE

Fatigue is a serious problem that needs to be addressed. Lack of energy affects vitality, emotions and personal relationships. In fact, it can affect your whole life and your happiness. Fatigue is both a symptom and a warning. It can be emotional, mental, spiritual, psychological or physical. Fatigue can stem from a multitude of conditions. Common causes are anemia, allergies, autointoxication, candida, Epstein-Barr virus, hypoglycemia, hypothyroidism, toxic metal poisoning, physical stress and lack of nutrients.

Fatigue or exhaustion cannot usually be dealt with by additional rest. There has to be a change in diet and thinking. Negative thinking has a profound detrimental effect on the body. Any type of stress can cause

❖

complete exhaustion. A person with a strong constitution can probably endure more stress than someone with a weak constitution, but it will eventually catch up with them. A sign of fatigue is that a person cannot cope with situations as he or she used to. Constant frustration and anger for no apparent reason are other signs of exhaustion and fatigue, as is loss of sexual desire. This is one reason people turn to drugs and stimulants is to try and recapture the energy they once had. I believe the underlying cause is lack of nutrients being assimilated in the body. Autointoxication and digestive problems are the main cause.

Natural Therapy: Fatigue is a symptom of a toxic body not assimilating nutrients necessary for energy. The blood needs to be purified with blood purifiers and the colon needs to be cleaned with lower bowel cleaners, enemas, or colonics. With a proper diet and cleansing program the body will gradually gain strength and energy. It may take months or years, but patience and a positive attitude will speed the healing. Begin exercising once you start gaining strength. The cells needs oxygen, so deep breathing will also bring energy to the cells. Stimulation through chiropractic treatments restores balance to the brain and nervous system. The brain has the knowledge to correct problems that exist in different areas of the body. Along with nutrition, health can be restored.

Foods to Heal: Fresh vegetables and steamed vegetables (contain minerals to prevent fatigue), fresh fruit and juices (cleansing and healing), whole grains, either slow or thermos cooking to retain nutrients (B-complex vitamins, enzymes and minerals), seeds (sesame, sunflower, pumpkin), nuts (almonds, pecans, filberts, and cashews).

Vitamins and Minerals: Take a multivitamin supplement (yeast free) with extra B$_6$, B$_{12}$ and pantothenic acid (promotes energy). Also supplement with vitamins C and E to get oxygen to the cells. Liquid multiminerals, extra calcium and magnesium (balance), chromium, iron, potassium, selenium and zinc are also beneficial.

Herbal Combinations: Anemia, blood purifier, bone (minerals), candida, digestion, energy, hypoglycemia, immune, lower bowels.

Single Herbs: Key herbs are capsicum, dong quai, ginkgo (strengthens the body) and ginseng, an energy booster that helps restore energy reserves by increasing carbohydrate metabolism and glycogen storage. Other important herbs are gotu kola (food for the brain), hawthorn, ho-shou-wu (tonic for the glands), licorice (provides energy and balances hormones), red clover (cleans blood for clearer thinking), schizandra (improves oxygen utilization and restores energy reserve) and suma (stimulates brain function). Other beneficial herbs are alfalfa, black cohosh, burdock, chaparral, dandelion, garlic, ginger, gentian (heals digestive system), goldenseal, hops (heals the nerves), lobelia, mistletoe, myrrh, skullcap (strengthens the brain and nerves), St. John's wort, valerian, wood betony, wormwood and yellow dock.

Supplements: Acidophilus, bee pollen, chlorophyll, herbal teas (oatstraw, red raspberry,), evening primrose oil, salmon oil, coenzyme Q_{10}, germanium, lecithin (quick energy to the brain).

Avoid: All stimulants that deplete the body of needed energy. Stay away from alcohol, tobacco and caffeine. Chocolate, soft drinks, candy and any sugar foods are stimulating to an already weakened body. Meat and processed food rob the body of vital nutrients.

✤ FIBROCYSTIC DISEASE (FEMALE)

Fibrocystic breast disease afflicts over 50 percent of adult females in the United States. This is a benign lump condition that rarely turns cancerous. In the past it was attributed to hormonal upset and is still regarded as such by many physicians. In a way it is a hormonal imbalance. Many health nutritionists believe that the problem stems from too much "unfavorable" estrogen, estradiol, a type of estrogen that the liver cannot filter because of congestion in the colon. This bad estrogen travels to the primary estrogen receptors of the body (especially in the breasts and uterus) and is responsible for proliferating tissue, which causes cysts and growths. Estradiol and other toxins back up into the blood stream and enter the breasts, brain or other parts of the body to cause lumps, congestion and other diseases in the system. When the liver is congested, it cannot filter harmful substances such as caffeine, found in coffee, tea, cola and chocolate.

Natural Therapy: A liver and lower bowel cleanse is essential and a high-fiber diet is beneficial. Changing dietary habits is necessary for a

❖

healthy liver to filter toxins that cause cysts, lumps and cancerous growths. Blood purification therapy will help the healing process. Avoid meat; it contains hormones (estrogen). Antibiotics increase the chances of breast lumps. The bowels must be kept active.

Foods to Heal: Almonds, sesame and sunflower seeds, raw fruits and green leafy vegetables and sprouts. A high-fiber diet using whole grains and vegetables will help prevent growths. Potassium foods are good because cysts and growths cannot live in a high potassium environment: dulse, kelp, Irish moss, lima beans, rice bran, whole grains, bananas, white and pinto beans, mung beans (sprouted), dried peas, apricots, pistachio nuts, peaches (dried), lentils, chickpeas, parsley and prunes. Fresh lemon juice in warm water will help cleanse the liver. Green drinks such as wheat grass juice will clean the blood and liver.

Vitamins and Minerals: Vitamin A protects the body from cancer-causing toxins and a deficiency contributes to growths. B-complex, (especially pantothenic acid, niacin, and riboflavin) protects against cysts and growths. The liver cannot eliminate estradiol without B vitamins, especially choline and inositol. B_6 is necessary to manufacture progesterone, an estrogen antagonist. B_{15} increases the body's resistance to oxygen deficiency (oxygen deficiency causes cancer and tumors to invade the cells). B vitamins are leached from the liver if too much sugar, processed starches and alcohol are present. Vitamin C neutralizes the damaging effect of carcinogenic material in food. Vitamin E, a powerful antioxidant, helps prevent fat oxidation and formation of free radicals which cause breast cancer. A multimineral is vital for a healthy body. Calcium and magnesium (found in herbs such as horsetail) are excellent in balancing minerals. Iodine (found in kelp) and zinc enhance the body's ability to make use of essential fatty acids. Selenium protects the body against toxins.

Herbal Combinations: Blood purifiers, digestion, glands, immune, lower bowels, nerve, potassium.

Single Herbs: Key herbs are burdock, chaparral, dandelion (cleans liver), echinacea (cleans glands), garlic, goldenseal, kelp, milk thistle, pau d'arco (protects liver from toxins), red clover (drink red clover blend teas), and yellow dock.

Supplements: Acidophilus (friendly bacteria), liquid chlorophyll, and lecithin. Evening primrose oil, salmon oil, or flaxseeds contain essential fatty acids.

Avoid: Sugar because it leaches B vitamins. Reduce fat intake—excess fat causes chronic diseases. Eliminate coffee, chocolate, tea and caffeine soft drinks as they contain harmful chemicals known as methylxanthines. Avoid alcohol and drugs; they destroy vitamins and minerals and promote fibrous growths and cysts. White flour products have no nutritional value and congest the liver and colon.

✦ FOOD POISONING

Food poisoning can be very serious if it isn't taken care of properly. Nature usually takes over and causes diarrhea and vomiting to rid the body of toxins. Symptoms of food poisoning include diarrhea, nausea, vomiting and cramps, lasting from a few hours to a few days. Twenty-four hours is the common duration. When it lasts longer, it is usually thought to be the flu.

The body has a natural way of dealing with poisons, toxins, worms, and parasites that enter our bodies. It naturally produces hydrochloric acid, which kills and destroys toxins and protects the digestive system. But, the typical American diet which is very high in sugar, white flour products, meat and fried oil, destroys the body's ability to produce this acid. Therefore, toxins can enter and cause us much distress.

There are many kinds of food poisoning: botulism, salmonella, *Staphylococcus aureus*, *Clostridium botulinum* ("cafeteria botulinum"), and giardiasis (associated with contaminated water).

Care must be taken in preparing food. If you use eggs, be very careful. They are susceptible to salmonella bacteria. Left-out potato salad can cause problems. Canned food with bulging tops should never be used. Use common sense when preparing and eating food and you can avoid food poisoning. Salmonella poisoning can be contracted from chicken, eggs, beef and pork products. Poorly cooked meat can cause this poison to thrive. Use chlorinated water after handling raw meat to protect against salmonella.

❖

Natural Therapy: Keep the blood clean and pure with blood purifier herbs. Using herbs that kill bacteria (goldenseal, garlic) will help keep the intestinal tract clean. Change to a natural diet, which will help prevent germs and bacteria from forming. Bacteria, germs and toxins will not live in a clean body.

Foods to Heal: Citrus juices diluted with pure water. Vegetable potassium broths (potato peelings, onions, garlic, parsley, celery as well as other vegetables, strain and drink the broth). Herbal teas soothe the stomach. After vomiting drink mint teas which will calm the stomach (peppermint, spearmint, catnip and chamomile, and alfalfa-mint tea are healing). Nature usually prevents you from being hungry, but if you are, don't eat; it will only stop the cleansing and drive the toxins further into the system where it will later cause chronic disease.

Vitamins and Minerals: Vitamin A (an emulsion enters the system faster) and liquid vitamin C with bioflavonoids (helps detoxify and strengthen the body). Take a multimineral because minerals are depleted quickly when vomiting, especially potassium. An herbal mineral formula is best.

Herbal Combinations: Blood purifiers, digestion, colds and flu, lower bowels, nerves, stress.

Single Herbs: Key herbs are catnip (calms the stomach), garlic (natural antibiotic), gentian (healing for the digestive system), ginger (calming for upset stomach), goldenseal (heals the digestive system), kelp (cleans and provides minerals) and red clover. Other important herbs are alfalfa, aloe vera (cleansing and healing), bayberry, black walnut (kills worms and parasites), buckthorn, burdock, capsicum, cascara sagrada, chaparral, dandelion, echinacea, ginseng, hawthorn, Irish moss, licorice, lobelia (cleans the stomach), myrrh, psyllium, watercress, yarrow, yellow dock.

Supplements: Free-form amino acids (enter system quickly for tissue repair), acidophilus (replaces friendly bacteria that is lost with diarrhea and vomiting), ipecac (induces vomiting), charcoal (absorbs toxins), and blue-green algae (cleans and repairs cells).

Avoid: All sugar products, fried foods, white flour products, meat, cheese, drugs; (will only weaken the body more). Stop eating. This is the best thing you can do so the body can heal itself the way nature intended.

❖ FRACTURES

There is good reason to take care of our bones. They are capable of supporting heavy loads and are a storehouse of calcium and other minerals. They are the seat of the vital red blood cells. Bones protect the delicate body parts and the joints that allows us to move about freely. But a broken bone can happen to anyone. Bones, even though they are strong, suffer weakness when injuries, genetic weakness, metabolic disorders, and aging take place. But they do not have to be weak if we take care in keeping them strong and healthy. It doesn't matter how old you get—your bones can repair themselves with proper nutrients. Bones are comprised of minerals, calcium and phosphorus deposited on a type of protein which is called collagen. Collagen formation requires vitamin C with bioflavonoids for healthy bones and connective tissues.

We can both prevent sports injuries such as runner's knee, tennis elbow, torn cartilage and ligaments, and broken or dislocated bones, and heal these injuries faster with a good diet that includes lots of minerals.

Natural Therapy: See a doctor for proper healing of bones to take place. Drink vegetable juices (carrot, celery, parsley), and vegetable broths. These, as well as fresh salads, contain a lot of minerals for healing. Herbs also contain a lot of minerals especially good for bone healing.

Foods to Heal: Broccoli, sprouted grains, kale leaves, parsley, carrot juice, whey powder, and homemade sauerkraut.

Vitamins and Minerals: Vitamin A is essential for healing and vital for protein assimilation. Vitamin C with bioflavonoids will speed the healing. B-vitamins speed healing. Vitamin D, along with calcium, is necessary for bone repair. Selenium and zinc will also expedite healing. Silicon, found in oatstraw and horsetail, is the king of bone healers. Calcium and magnesium are essential for bone healing. (I prefer the herbal calcium formulas.) Potassium and sodium balance will help keep the swelling under control. Trace minerals such as copper, manganese and zinc are important for bone formation.

Herbal Combinations: Bone formulas, digestion, lower bowel, potassium, nerves (help keep the pain under control).

Single Herbs: Key herbs are alfalfa (rich in minerals), aloe vera (healing and cleansing), capsicum, comfrey (promotes bone healing), dande-

❖

lion, garlic, gentian, goldenseal (cleans the digestive tract), hops (helps in pain), horsetail (repairs bones with rich silicon content), kelp (rich in minerals), skullcap (helps relax muscles), wood betony (acts as a tranquilizer) and yellow dock. Other beneficial herbs are black cohosh, burdock, chaparral, dong quai, ginseng, gotu kola, hawthorn, lobelia, mistletoe.

Supplements: Blue-green algae (increases healing), liquid chlorophyll, flaxseed (essential fatty acids) and liquid minerals for faster assimilation. Use hydrochloric acid and pancreatic enzymes for assimilation of minerals.

Avoid: All sugar products (they leach calcium from bones), caffeine, and cola drinks. White flour products are void of B-vitamins and minerals. Chocolate leaches calcium and B-vitamins from bones.

❖ GOUT

The tendency for gout can be hereditary but it doesn't mean you have to be plagued by this ailment. Too much uric acid in the blood and tissues causes gout. It crystallizes in the joints and creates swelling and pain from the abrasive action of the uric acid crystals. Attacks can occur in the night with pain in the joint of the big toe. It is usually swollen, red and tender to the touch. Wrist, ankle or thumb joints may be affected. Gout has been associated with drinking beer, wine and a high-meat diet.

Natural Therapy: Blood purification and colon cleanse will help this ailment. Foot reflexology will help break up the crystals, and blood purifiers (herbal) will help eliminate the crystals out of the body. Foot reflexology may be painful but worth it to get rid of this painful ailment.

Foods to Heal: Raw vegetable juices (carrot, celery, parsley) and green drinks are rich in chlorophyll. Drink unsweetened cherry juice. Make vegetable broths, using potato peelings, celery with leaves, onions, parsley, and other vegetables. Strain and drink the broth because it contains potassium and other minerals to dissolve uric acid deposits.

Vitamins and Minerals: Vitamin A prevents toxins from accumulating in joints, B-complex vitamins aid in metabolism, vitamin C with bioflavonoids eliminates uric acid from blood, and vitamin E increases circulation and destroys free radicals. Multiminerals eliminate uric acid and create healing. Selenium and zinc help in tissue repair and healing bones.

Herbal Combinations: Arthritis formulas, blood purifiers, bone, digestion, nerve and pain formulas.

Single Herbs: Alfalfa, aloe vera, burdock (blood purifier), capsicum (helps in circulation), chaparral (cleans blood and uric acid), comfrey (healing), dandelion (cleans liver to filter uric acid), devil's claw (cleanses vascular walls, and eliminates toxin from the blood), dulse (rich in minerals), garlic, hydrangea (helps kidneys to eliminate uric acid), kelp, parsley, papaya, saffron, red clover, watercress, white willow and yucca (anti-stress properties).

Supplements: Free-form amino acids, cystine (works with pantothenic acid in gout treatment), histidine (removes heavy metals and toxins), phenylalanine (for pain). Distilled water, green drinks, coenzyme Q_{10}, fish oil lipids, salmon oil, evening primrose oil, Chinese essential oils and tea tree oil (for external use).

Avoid: All meats are very high in uric acid. White flour and sugar products only increases the ailment. Rich foods such as cakes, pies, ice cream, candy only irritate the problem. Sardines, high salt diet, organ meats, meat gravies and broths will aggravate gout.

✣ Hair Health

Beautiful hair adds to a person's attractiveness but it also has practical purposes. It conserves body heat, protects the scalp and it plays a role in the sensory system. The hair follicles, which are at the root of each hair shaft, are surrounded by sensory nerves that react whenever the hair shaft is touched or brushed.

The hair shaft is the part that grows above the skins surface. It is alive and is affected by hormones, enzymes, blood, perspiration, environment and genetics. The use of dyes, chemicals, permanents, and some shampoos are hard on the hair, not to mention the dust, air pollution and chemicals in the air. Hair dyes contain harmful chemicals and not only penetrate the scalp but dry out the hair. The dyes can also enter the blood stream and cause adverse reactions in the body. Lead in the products is only one problem that arises from using hair dyes.

❖

Dietary deficiency is something we can change to improve our hair health. It seems to be the last thing we think about when we have dull, receding hairlines, bald spots or undue loss of hair. The idea that nutritional deficiencies may be showing up in the conditions of the hair does not dawn on us, but nutrition is key in having healthy hair. Hair analysis is an effective tool to determine what is lacking in the body or what there is too much of. Toxic metal measured by hair analysis are cadmium, lead, arsenic, mercury and aluminum to name a few. Minerals are about 200 times more concentrated in the hair than they are in the blood, making them easier to measure accurately. Hair analysis reflects concentrations of toxic metals, revealing the buildup of these elements in the tissues. It will help determine mineral deficiencies in the body.

Natural Therapy: Blood purification, cleansing fasts and fresh vegetable juices (rich in minerals). Stimulation therapy will help cleanse and bring nutrients to the scalp area. Olive oil and wheat germ oil are good for scalp stimulation. Hot and cold towels, alternating each for about twelve minutes will bring circulation to the head area. A colon cleanse will also help rid the body of toxins that contribute to hair loss. Make certain digestion is efficient enough for mineral assimilation. Exercise helps to relax the entire body and mind and it increases circulation. The hair follicles need circulation for nourishment through the blood to stimulate hair growth.

Foods to Heal: Herbal teas that help are rosemary, sage, nettle and oatstraw. Raw and steamed vegetables contain minerals essential for hair health. Whole grains contain B vitamins for healthy hair. The protein found in grains, seeds, and nuts is essential for healthy hair because hair is 95 to 98 percent protein. A variety of whole grains (thermos cooking) and fruits and vegetables will improve the general condition of the hair.

Vitamins and Minerals: Vitamin A protects against dry scalp, which can cause baldness. It is also good for liver function and an unhealthy liver can result in hair loss. B-complex vitamins are essential for healthy hair; lack of B$_1$ can cause gray hair and hair loss. This vitamin helps in digestion, assimilation and elimination of food. Lack of B$_2$ causes dull hair and loss of hair. B$_6$ and pantothenic acid are good for gray hair; a deficiency causes excessively oily skin and hair. B_{12} acts as a nutritional stimulant to prevent gray hair, loss of hair and dry scaly skin. Biotin and choline and inositol work together to protect hair follicles. Vitamin C with bioflavonoids protects the immune system and works with B_{12} in the breakdown and utilization of protein. PABA and pantothenic acid help increase hair growth and natural · color. Vitamin E improves circulation and helps to balance hormones which can cause hair loss. All minerals are essential for healthy hair. Silicon and sulphur are essential for new hair growth. Calcium normalizes mineral metabolism. Chlorine, copper and fluorine work with silicon for healthy hair. Iodine, iron, magnesium, manganese, potassium and zinc are also important.

Herbal Combinations: Blood purifier, bone, female problems formulas to balance hormones, gland, hair-skin-nail, nerve, stress.

Single Herbs: Key herbs are alfalfa (rich in minerals), black cohosh (balances hormones), dulse (rich in minerals), horsetail (rich in silicon), jojoba oil (cleans and nourishes the scalp), kelp (rich in minerals), licorice (helps adrenals), oatstraw (rich in silicon), parsley, rosemary and yarrow. Other important herbs are comfrey, pau d'arco, red clover, red raspberry, sarsaparilla, slippery elm, watercress and wormwood.

Supplements: Essential fatty acids (a lack of can cause hair to fall out), salmon oil, evening primrose oil, lecithin, blue-green algae, rice bran syrup, chelated cell salts.

Avoid: Refined sugars and white flour products, rancid oils, ham, bacon, hot dogs, corned beef, lunch meats, alcohol, processed foods, fried foods and salt. These foods create stress on the body and deplete nutrients rapidly.

❖ HALITOSIS (BAD BREATH)

Bad breath can be caused from diseased teeth or gums, chronically infected tonsils, sinuses or nasal infections, or even lung abscess and bronchial disease. The main cause of bad breath is constipation. The residue from food that is not digested properly can ferment and rot in the intestines, producing an odor. Lack of hydrochloric acid in the stomach and lack of the normal mucus coating of the stomach can also cause odors, especially in the elderly. Regular bowel function is essential to avoid accumulation of waste and toxin products which can reabsorb into the bloodstream and disrupt the chemistry of the gastrointestinal tract. In the morning, when the valves of the stomach are open, the smell is most prevalent.

Natural Therapy: Blood purification and bowel cleansing therapy are needed. Cleansing the intestinal tract for better absorption and elimination will improve bad breath. If the lungs are the problem, deep breathing exercises will help clean the bottom of the lungs which are not always thoroughly cleansed. Chewing whole cloves and parsley will also help bad breath.

Foods to Heal: A cleansing diet using all raw foods, especially raw fruit and vegetable juices, is recommended.

Vitamins and Minerals: Vitamins A, B-complex, C with bioflavonoids and E will heal and protect against toxins accumulating in the body. A multimineral supplement with extra potassium, selenium and zinc is also beneficial.

Herbal Combinations: Blood purifier, digestion, liver, lower bowels.

Single Herbs: Key herbs are alfalfa, aloe vera (cleans the digestive tract), cascara sagrada (cleans and strengthens the bowels), cloves (sweetens the breath and helps in digestion), kelp (rich in minerals), goldenseal (cleans the digestive tract for better assimilation), parsley (destroys odors) and peppermint (sweetens the breath and helps in digestion). Other vital herbs are chaparral, echinacea, Irish moss, myrrh and watercress.

Supplements: Liquid chlorophyll, acidophilus, green drinks, fresh lemon juice in pure water, blue-green algae.

Avoid: Constipation, which will not only cause bad breath, but create other diseases. Avoid all unnatural food: sugar (not a food), salt, meat, especially salted and preserved with additives. White flour products.

✧ HAY FEVER

Millions of Americans suffer untold allergic reactions each spring and summer. They manifest themselves in watery, itching eyes, runny nose, blurred vision, headaches, sinus aches and pains and a head that feels as big as a balloon.

❖

A common type of allergy is hay fever, an inflammation of the nasal mucosa. Healthy mucous membranes protect all the organ linings from invasion by bacteria; when the mucous membranes are not healthy, they are vulnerable to irritation by germs or any airborne irritant, and this irritation results in an increase of mucus flow which is out of control. Red, swollen eyes, tickling in the nose and throat, and difficulty in breathing are common symptoms of hay fever. It usually continues day after day, growing worse year after year, unless natural methods are used to treat it.

Hay fever and all other allergic reactions are the body's attempt to try to clean and purify itself of toxins. Long before hay fever develops there is catarrh of the stomach due to an abuse of overloading the stomach with overeating the wrong combinations and wrong kinds of food. It could also stem from too much rich food. We build up protein and starch acids which create other acids from the overconsumption of fried and rancid oils. These all cause irritations and inflammations of the stomach lining, leading to a chronic gastric fermentation. Resulting gas is passed directly by way of the stomach to the lungs, where it builds up. Conditions such as hay fever are primarily caused by the irritations from gas elimination that is being generated in the stomach.

When the body is overloaded with too many toxins and trying to eliminate them from the natural eliminative organs (the kidneys, colon or skin), the stress is then put on the lungs and nasal membranes. In trying to eliminate chronic catarrh, hay fever develops. It may take years of the accumulation of toxins before hay fever develops, or it can start from birth with toxins inherited from the parents.

Natural Therapy: Blood purification therapy is needed to clean and strengthen the body. Cleaning the blood and lower bowels will speed up the elimination of hay fever. Skin brushing will help eliminate gas and toxins from the skin. Foot reflexology and chiropractic treatments will speed circulation and healing.

Foods to Heal: Green drinks will help purify the blood. Raw diet and proper food combining will help in assimilation and elimination of food. Raw vegetable salads with sprouts, sprouted grains, wheat grass juice, barley green drinks and fresh fruit are cleansers of the body. Do short fasts using citrus juices as they are very cleansing.

❖

Vitamins and Minerals: Vitamin A protects and heals the mucous membranes. B-vitamins are depleted quickly in acute diseases. Pantothenic acid is essential in the production of cortisone. Vitamin C with bioflavonoids has a natural antihistamine effect. Vitamin F helps suppress the release of histamines and prevents fluid accumulation outside the blood vessels. A multimineral supplement is good because all minerals are essential for healing the body. Selenium, silicon and zinc are all necessary for healing.

Herbal Combinations: Allergy blood purifiers, bone, digestion, lungs, lower bowels.

Single Herbs: Key herbs are burdock (cleans blood), cayenne (improves circulation), chaparral (cleans and eliminates toxins), chickweed (soothing and healing for the respiratory system), comfrey (cleans up dead tissues and restores new), echinacea (builds up the immune system), fenugreek (dissolves hardened mucus and expels toxins), goldenseal (a natural antibiotic and healer), licorice (induces the adrenal glands to produce their own natural cortisone, provides strength to a weakened system), lobelia (cleans the stomach), ma huang (a natural antihistamine), marshmallow (contains antiseptic properties and is healing and soothing), myrrh, pau d'arco (cleans liver for better elimination of toxins), red raspberry, skullcap, slippery elm (high in nutrients such as calcium, zinc and vitamin C, and is healing) and yellow dock. Other important herbs are alfalfa, aloe vera, dandelion (protects the liver), eyebright, gentian (heals the digestive tract), hops, Irish moss, wood betony and wormwood.

Supplements: Bee pollen, acidophilus (milk free), blue-green algae, essential fatty acids such as salmon oil, evening primrose oil and fish lipids.

Avoid: Milk and milk products create extra mucus, and meat contains hormones, additives and antibiotics that create irritations. Wheat may sometimes cause problems since it may not be digesting, so use millet, brown rice, buckwheat or corn meal instead. Avoid white sugar products—they deplete vitamins and minerals necessary for strengthening mucous membranes.

❖ HEADACHES (ALSO MIGRAINES)

In 1932, in *Medical Journal and Record,* a doctor wrote, "Headaches are among the most frequent complaints of human life." Today headaches are still one of the most common complaints doctors see. It is commonly believed that headaches are the price we pay for fast-paced living, but it isn't true. Headaches are as old as recorded history and were as common in primitive societies as they are today. In ancient Melanesian, European and MesoAmerican societies, it was believed that puncturing the skull (called trephining) to free evil spirits would cure persistent headaches, epilepsy or insanity. Skulls with trephining punctures go back ages to the Neolithic and Bronze ages.

An estimated 80 million Americans will suffer from headache pain and about 10 million will be afflicted with migraine. Thirty million pounds of aspirin are consumed each year in the United States. Headaches are a symptom, not a disease. They are a result of dietary habits, lifestyle, environment, tension in the neck, shoulders or back, sinus problems, and, less commonly, from brain tumors.

Autointoxication headaches are the most common and, in the opinion of many health oriented doctors, originate from the stomach. Wrong food combinations, overeating and junk food will cause fermentation in the intestines and stomach. This causes gas, which enters the blood and causes irritation on the nerves and brain and causes headaches. Pressure in the temples and forehead usually indicate that there are stomach problems. Throbbing pain often results from congestion in the liver, spleen or digestive tract. Migraine headaches are caused by excess starches and sugars in the diet.

If the stomach, colon and mucous membranes were healthy, then allergic reactions to food wouldn't cause headaches. Stress, tension, constipation, sinusitis, head injury, air pollution, poor circulation and poor respiration are all causes of headaches. Allergies to MSG, chocolate, caffeine, wheat (pesticides), sulfites, sugar, dairy products, alcohol and vinegar can also cause headaches. An emotional conflict or anxiety can cause real headaches. High blood pressure can cause headaches. Children with headaches often have eye problems, but they could be caused by allergies, or emotions.

Natural Therapy: Blood purifiers and lower bowel cleansers. Chiropractic treatments and foot reflexology will help normal nerve stimulation.

❖

bones may be out of place. Tension in the jaws, neck or head can he helped by manipulation. Change to a natural diet using fresh vegetables and fruits. Eat whole grains, cooked thermos style for retention of B-vitamins and enzymes. A cool cloth on the neck and head will relieve some headaches, while rest and relaxation will help others.

Foods to Heal: Herbal teas such as chamomile, mint and ginger, and pure water. Detoxify the body with fresh vegetable juices for healing and fruit juices for cleansing. Use wheat grass juice, green drinks. Change to a wholesome diet using grains, beans, fresh salads, steamed vegetables, seeds nuts and sprouts. They are healing and nourishing to the body.

Vitamins and Minerals: Vitamin A heals the mucous membranes, B-complex with extra niacin, B_{15} and pangamic acid will relax muscles. A deficiency of vitamin B_5 (pantothenic acid) results in headaches and depression. Vitamin C with bioflavonoids constricts and cleans veins, and E increases oxygen in the blood. Take a multimineral with extra calcium and magnesium (balance), potassium, iron and iodine. Zinc can give headache relief, and all minerals are vital for health.

Herbal Combinations: Allergy blood purifier, digestion, glands, lower bowels, nerve, pain and stress formulas.

Single Herbs: Key herbs are burdock (a blood purifier), cascara sagrada, chamomile, dandelion (liver cleanser), feverfew, goldenseal (helps clean the digestive tract where headaches can originate), hops (relaxes nerves, calms pain), horsetail (rich in minerals), psyllium (cleans the colon), red clover (excellent blood cleanser), skullcap (helps in pain), white willow (pain reliever) and wood betony (relieves pain). Other important herbs are alfalfa, aloe vera, black cohosh, black walnut, buchu, buckthorn, capsicum, chaparral, echinacea, garlic, ginger, ginseng, hawthorn, ho-shou-wu, licorice, St. John's wort, uva ursi, yarrow, yellow dock and yucca.

Supplements: Lecithin, rice bran syrup and evening primrose oil. Externally, use Chinese essential oils, tea tree oil, salmon oil, spirulina, blue-green algae.

Avoid: Constipation, wrong food combining, MSG, nitrates and nitrites used to preserve or cure meats, nicotine and caffeine. Tyramine is a food chemical that dilates blood vessels and can cause headaches. Foods containing tyramine are aged cheeses, pickled herring, salted

❖

and dried fish, sausages, beef and chicken, liver, sauerkraut, vanilla, chocolate, yeast, some soy sauce, beer, ale and red wines.

❖ HEMORRHOIDS (VARICOSE VEINS)

Hemorrhoids and varicose veins are caused by chronic constipation and circulatory system weakness. Liver congestion has been implicated as another cause. It occurs as a result of pregnancy, junk food diet (clogs the circulatory system), lack of exercise, sitting while working, heavy lifting and obesity. It is also seen in low-fiber diets.

Varicose veins occur most often in the legs. Weakness in the veins allows blood to accumulate and stretch the capillaries and veins, causing discoloration, tenderness and sometimes pain.

There are external hemorrhoids and internal hemorrhoids. External are easily identifiable and usually more painful. Internal hemorrhoids may be present for years and not cause trouble. They can also appear externally if they become swollen and protrude the anal ring. Bleeding may be the first sign of internal hemorrhoids. Constant bleeding over a period of time can cause anemia. If left untreated, varicose veins can lead to phlebitis, leg ulcers, permanently swollen legs, pulmonary emboli, and even surface leg hemorrhaging.

Natural Therapy: Blood purification, circulatory strengthening and lower bowel cleansers will help in hemorrhoids and varicose veins. Liver cleansing promotes a better filtering of toxins. A high-fiber diet, using whole grains, fresh salads and vegetables strengthens the veins. Use sprouted seeds and grains, and fresh fruits. Use short fasts, using green drinks, wheat grass juice and pure water. Carrot and celery juices are also beneficial. Exercise—even simple walking—will strengthen veins and increase circulation. It will also help prevent deposits of clotting blood within the veins. Raw red potato or clove of garlic can be used several times a week as a suppository for hemorrhoids. Sitz baths, continued for several days, will help strengthen veins. A sitz bath involves using two basins, one with hot water, one with cold. Use the hot basin first and cold last. The warm water relaxes the spasms of the muscles and the cold tightens the tissues.

Foods to Heal: Figs, raisins and prunes, soaked in pure water before eat-

❖

ing. Citrus fruit, using the inner skin, will strengthen and heal veins. Okra, rich in silicon and selenium, helps opens clogged veins and strengthen capillaries. Oat bran is very beneficial for keeping the veins clean. Buckwheat contains rutin, a bioflavonoid that strengthens the veins and decreases the tendency of the capillaries to break easily.

Vitamins and Minerals: Vitamin A strengthens the veins. Take B-complex vitamins with extra B_6, B_{12}, B_{15}, choline and inositol (found in lecithin). Vitamin C with bioflavonoids strengthens the veins and capillaries. Vitamin E is a vital nutrient for varicose veins because it protects the cells and veins from damage. Also apply vitamin E externally. A multimineral supplement with extra silicon and selenium will open up clogged veins and strengthen them. Zinc, calcium and vitamin D are very important in healing veins.

Herbal Combinations: Blood purifier, bone, chelation (cleans the veins), colitis, digestion, liver and gallbladder, lower bowels.

Single Herbs: Key herbs are aloe vera, black walnut (rich in minerals), butcher's broom (strengthens the blood vessels and keeps them clean), capsicum, cascara sagrada (colon rebuilder), comfrey, goldenseal, horsetail (contains silicon), kelp (strengthens and cleans veins), mullein oil (relieves pain), oatstraw, pau d'arco (cleans the liver and protects the system), white oak bark (strengthens veins) and witch hazel. Other vital herbs are alfalfa, bayberry, buckthorn, chaparral, lobelia, parsley, red raspberry, slippery elm, uva ursi and wood betony.

Supplements: Bee pollen, blue-green algae, glucomannan, lecithin, liquid chlorophyll, oak bark poultice, psyllium, spirulina, salmon oil, germanium, and coenzyme Q_{10}. Use a liquid mineral and herb drinks. Comfrey and goldenseal ointment and calendula ointment help with itching and pain; mullein oil also helps in pain. Wheat grass poultices will stimulate healing of tissues. Clay packs will stimulate healing.

Avoid: Margarine and all unnatural fats, meat (especially beef), high sugar foods, and white flour.

❖ HEPATITIS (LIVER PROBLEMS, JAUNDICE)

The liver is the largest solid organ in the body, weighing about four pounds, and is the detoxifier of the body. Everything we eat, drink, breathe and absorb through the skin is purified by the liver. Thousands of chemical reactions take place in the liver every second of our lives. Eighty percent of the liver can be destroyed and it will still keep us alive. Some of the functions of the liver are:

1. Controlling the production and elimination of cholesterol.
2. Maintaining hormone balance.
3. Regulating blood clotting.
4. Helping the body resist infection by producing immune factors and removing bacteria from the bloodstream.
5. Maintaining and monitoring the proper level of many chemicals and drugs in the blood.
6. Cleansing the blood and discharging waste products into the bile.
7. Neutralizing and destroying poisonous substances.
8. Regulating fat distribution.
9. Metabolizing alcohol.
10. Aiding the digestive process by producing bile.
11. Producing quick energy when it is needed.
12. Storing iron and other vitamins, minerals and sugars to prevent shortages when it is needed.
13. Manufacturing new body proteins.
14. It has the ability to regenerate its own damaged tissue.

The medical term for hepatitis is "inflammation of the liver." There are two types of hepatitis—A and B. Hepatitis A is a viral infection and is transmitted by saliva, semen, urine or fecal contamination of water or food. Hepatitis B, or serum hepatitis, is mainly transmitted in hospitals by needles used for drugs, transfusions and dialysis.

Toxic overload is the basic cause of liver problems. Our bodies can tolerate a certain amount of contamination, but when the liver is overloaded, toxins will circulate in the blood and enter the brain, nervous system or other organs, and interfere with the normal functioning. Constipation is the main cause of overload of the liver. When the liver tries to expel the poisons forced on it, the kidneys become burdened, for it is through the kidneys that the impurities are ultimately expelled. Some of the signs of liver malfunction are: yellowed complexion, digestive disturbances, sluggish feeling in the mornings, headaches (the direct cause is constipation) and insomnia.

❖

Natural Therapy: Blood purification, liver purifiers and lower bowel therapy. The liver handles whatever we eat, so we need to protect it by giving it living food. Rest the liver with pure water and juice fasting. Use fresh lemon juice in warm water for a few days, fasting to restore liver function. Overeating is very hard on the liver. Lack of exercise can indirectly damage the liver by failing to stimulate the lungs to detoxify, causing an overburdened liver.

Foods to Heal: Lemon juice and celery juice with a little carrot juice are rich in vitamin A for healing. Beet juice is also healing. Eat a lot of green vegetables and sprouts, steamed vegetables, potassium broths (potato peelings, onions, carrot tops, celery), unsweetened yogurt, raw seeds and nuts, swiss chard, beet greens and celery. Strawberries, grapes and cherries are a tonic. Cold-pressed olive oil is cleansing and digestible for the liver. Grapefruit, oranges and avocados have a good influence on the liver. Eat mostly raw foods. Eating overcooked foods places a strain on the liver as they do not supply live enzymes and amino acids vital for proper digestion.

Vitamins and Minerals: Beta carotene has to convert to vitamin A in the liver, which puts a strain on it. B-complex vitamins are essential for a healthy liver: B_2 and B_6 for the breakdown and utilization of carbohydrates, fats and protein, and pantothenic and folic acid to fight stress. Use a vitamin B liquid, or injections if necessary. A deficiency of vitamin C can cause severe liver degeneration; it protects the liver from damage. Vitamin E speeds healing and prevents scarring, common in advanced stages of cirrhosis. Take a multimineral with extra calcium and magnesium (use herbal calcium), which are essential for blood clotting.

Herbal Combinations: Kidney liver and gallbladder formulas, digestion, lower bowels.

Single Herbs: Key herbs are burdock (restores function of liver and gallbladder), cascara sagrada (heals liver), dandelion (clears obstruction of the liver and detoxifies), gentian (a bitter herb that helps digestion and liver function), goldenseal (helps regulate liver function), licorice (combines well with bitter herbs to balance formulas), milk thistle (heals damaged liver), pau d'arco (protects the liver from further damage, strengthens the whole body), parsley and watercress (help keep liver in balance), saffron (digests fats to aid the liver and gall-bladder), wild yam (removes toxic buildup of bile), wormwood (stimulates the liver, eliminates worms) and yellow dock (rich in iron for a healthy liver).

Supplements: Blue-green algae, chlorophyll, germanium, coenzyme Q10, bentonite, evening primrose oil, salmon oil, and lecithin.

Avoid: Drugs are hard on the liver, especially sleeping pills. Avoid all fried foods, refined foods, sugars and artificial sweeteners and caffeine drinks. Avoiding eating too much—it overburdens the liver. Artificial colorings, preservatives, flavorings and other chemicals overwork the liver. Devitalized food clogs the liver, causes impure blood and irritates the stomach and intestines.

❖ HIATAL HERNIA

Hiatal hernia is a very common disease estimated to affect 50 percent of people over the age of forty. A hiatal hernia occurs when the small hole in the diaphragm that allows the esophagus to pass through to the stomach weakens and enlarges, allowing a portion of the stomach to protrude upward through the hole beside the esophagus. Leakage of acid in the lower esophagus often causes discomfort and a burning feeling.

A hiatal hernia can be caused by a low-fiber diet, straining due to constipation, lack of exercise, obesity, loss of muscle tone in stomach, or eating wrong combinations of food, causing fermentation and gas that protrudes the stomach upwards. Symptoms are the regurgitation of food, nausea, lack of appetite, intestinal gas, constipation and vomiting. Many people sleep with pillows under their head to alleviate the condition. Others sleep in a recliner to get relief. Some people have surgery but this does not help the cause of hiatal hernia. The cause needs to be treated naturally for permanent relief.

If a hiatal hernia isn't corrected, it can cause serious problems because of improper digestion and assimilation. Ulcers are also common with hiatal hernia, as are migraine headaches. A hiatal hernia affects the liver and creates problems with cholesterol that cannot be eliminated properly.

Theodore A. Baroody, Jr., D.C., provides a simple procedure that can help with hiatal hernia: "If there is shortness of breath, or the feeling that food is hung up and isn't going down properly, simply drink two 8-

ounce glasses of water and bounce on the heels 12 times. First, this puts weight in the stomach, then the bouncing will jar it into place." His book, *Hiatal Hernia Syndrome: Insidious Link To Major Illness,* gives valuable information on self-healing.

Natural Therapy: A chiropractor can manipulate a hiatal hernia back where it belongs. Blood purifiers, and lower bowel cleansers will help purify and clean the system. A proper diet is essential, as is proper food combining to avoid fermentation and formation of gas and toxins. Keep meals small and simple. Exercise will also help this ailment. Avoid using liquids with meals; they dilute hydrochloric acid which is essential in digestion of food. A loving, positive attitude is a must for a healthy stomach.

Foods to Heal: Eat raw nuts (almonds), seeds (sesame, sunflower, pumpkin), and figs and raisins (soak first). You can also soak nuts to make milk drinks. Healing fruits are apples, grapes, plums, peaches, bananas, and pineapple. Good, unsweetened juices are apple, cranberry, cherry and raspberry. Eat vegetables such as asparagus, avocados, beets, broccoli, cabbage, cauliflower, carrots, celery, cucumbers, peas, radishes, squash, string beans and tomatoes. Potatoes are good, either raw or baked. Brown rice, millet and buckwheat are healing and easy to digest.

Vitamins and Minerals: Vitamin A is very healing. B-complex vitamins are essential for a healthy stomach and digestion. Vitamin C with bioflavonoids is healing and cleansing. Multiminerals with extra calcium and magnesium, potassium, sodium (in herbs), selenium, silicon and zinc are healing.

Herbal Combinations: Blood purifiers, bone (rich in minerals), colitis formulas, digestion, glands, immune formulas, lower bowels, nerve and ulcer formulas.

Single Herbs: Key herbs are alfalfa, aloe vera (healing), capsicum, (healing and creates circulation), comfrey and pepsin, gentian (healing and strengthening for digestive system), ginger, goldenseal (excellent for healing), hops, horsetail, marshmallow, papaya, skullcap, slippery elm (healing and provides needed protein). Other helpful herbs are black walnut, burdock, echinacea, garlic, hawthorn, yellow dock and yucca.

--- ❖ ---

Supplements: Blue-green algae, liquid chlorophyll, and aloe vera juice (use a combination of comfrey, goldenseal, slippery elm and aloe vera mixed with apple juice and drink slowly for healing). Coenzyme Q_{10}, germanium, evening primrose oil, salmon oil, glucomannan and lecithin are also beneficial supplements.

Avoid: Alcohol, soft drinks, all sugar products, all caffeine drinks, and refined white-flour products such as spaghetti, macaroni, noodles and white rice.

❖ HERPES (SIMPLEX AND GENITAL HERPES)

Herpes Type I is called simplex and is recognized as cold sores and skin eruptions. They are most common on the mouth, lips, and in the eyes. Herpes Type II is genital herpes and is sexually transmitted and very contagious. The herpes II virus in pregnant women increases the chance of premature delivery or miscarriage. The baby could also be infected. It can cause brain, blindness or neurological damage. Herpes is a virus that is originally caused by skin-to-skin contact. It can lay dormant and than recur when the immune system is weakened through stress, diet, autointoxication, a feverish illness, overexposure to sunlight, or some foods and drugs. The initial infection can go away, but the virus often does not. Herpes hangs on, lodging itself in a dormant state in the skin or nervous system.

The type I virus usually starts with a brief period of itching or tingling, when you realize what you have. Small blisters will then appear and persist for several days before they begin to dry, forming a yellowish crust. Healing takes about a week to ten days, and maybe even three weeks. With natural treatment, herpes can be healed in a shorter period.

Natural Therapy: Blood purification and nervine therapy, also lower bowel cleansing. A cleansing diet is essential to restore the body to its normal balance. Use more alkaline foods to start with. Too much acid food will trigger herpes. Herpes is nature's method of cleansing impurities from the system for a healthier lifestyle. Don't suppress herpes; use natural remedies to eliminate the virus. Short fasts, using fresh vegetable juices will help. Daily exercise in the fresh air will build the immune system and increase resistance to disease. Learning to deal with stress and have a calm, loving attitude without anger, frustration and hate will also help.

Foods to Heal: Whole grains (thermos cooking), beans and steamed vegetables, fresh fruit, vegetables and sprouts, fresh fish, canned fish, chicken, and goat's milk. Food combining is very important. Drink pure water, vegetable and fruit juices, and herbal teas. Limit protein, especially red meat; it is very hard to digest. Chewing food well is easier on the digestive system and ensures better healing and building.

Vitamins and Minerals: Vitamin A is essential for healing the mucous membranes. Vitamin C with bioflavonoids is also healing, as are B-complex vitamins (yeast free). Vitamin E is healing. Multiminerals with extra calcium and magnesium (herbal calcium), selenium and zinc are healing and protects the immune system.

Herbal Combinations: Blood purifiers, bone, candida, colitis, digestion, immune, infection formulas, and lower bowel and stress formulas.

Single Herbs: Aloe vera (fresh and powdered), black walnut (external and internal), comfrey, garlic, goldenseal (heals), myrrh, Oregon grape, pau d'arco (cleans blood), red clover, rose hips and slippery elm (heals mucous membranes).

Supplements: Acidophilus, blue-green algae, evening primrose oil, salmon oil, lecithin, spirulina, tea tree oil (external), L-lysine.

Avoid: Chocolate, corn, peanuts and walnuts (all nuts can trigger herpes). Avoid alcohol, processed foods, all white sugar and white flour products, and caffeine drinks, both sodas and coffee.

✦ HIGH BLOOD PRESSURE (HYPERTENSION)

Hypertension is a disease that involves the heart and the arteries that carry fresh blood to every part of the body. It occurs when cholesterol deposits in the walls of the arteries harden and constrict the blood vessels, compressing the blood into a smaller volume and thereby raising its pressure. Hypertension is also manifested neurologically when emotional stress triggers the "fight or flight" response causing the muscles to squeeze these tiny blood vessels; they compress the blood into a smaller volume, which then raises the pressure.

Hypertension is a major killer that causes stroke, heart disease, kidney disease and other problems. It is a degenerative disease caused by incorrect living habits, eating and attitude towards living. We need to understand why we act the way we do. We need to deal with stress and tensions in our lives, but the body needs to be fortified nutritionally first, before we can even think properly. Strengthening the nervous system should be the first priority when dealing with stress.

Hypertension can be reversed only if we take control of our lives and change our eating and living habits. It is necessary to exercise more, watch our weight, and avoid alcohol, tobacco and drugs of all kinds. Chiropractic treatment is a way to determine if there is a pinched nerve or subluxation that might interfere with circulation and proper nerve function.

Natural Therapy: Blood purification, lower bowel therapy and nervine therapy will help in blood pressure. Short fasts using celery, parsley and cucumber juices will help reduce high blood pressure. If you have high blood pressure, doctors usually put you on diuretics immediately, and parsley is a natural diuretic. Exercise also helps to reduce the body's reaction to nervous stress. A combination of diet changes and exercise will show an improvement quickly.

Foods to Heal: High-fiber foods (whole grains, oat bran, beans, peas, vegetables and fruits) are healing. Potassium-rich foods are fruits, vegetables and unsalted nuts, green leafy vegetables, potatoes skins, bananas, oranges, sunflower seeds, nuts and raw garlic. Also good are lentils, oatmeal, brown rice and whole grain pasta.

Vitamins and Minerals: Take a multivitamin with extra A, C with bioflavonoids, K, and E (start slowly). Also necessary is a multimineral with extra calcium (herbal formulas); magnesium, manganese, silicon, selenium, sodium (natural) and zinc. Potassium and sodium will help reduce high blood pressure and avoid cardiovascular disease.

Herbal Combinations: Heart and blood pressure formulas, glands, nerves, bone combination, chelation, digestion, lower bowel.

Single Herbs: Key herbs are garlic (lowers blood pressure), hawthorn (strengthens the veins), hops (relaxes veins and nerves), passionflower (nerve relaxer), parsley (natural diuretic), pau d'arco (blood cleanser), skullcap (calms the nerves) and valerian (relaxer). Other vital herbs are alfalfa, aloe vera, black cohosh, capsicum (cleans the veins), dandelion (cleans the liver), echinacea (helps eliminate toxins from the veins), ginger, ginseng (strengthens the body), gotu kola (feeds the brain), lady's slipper, mistletoe, yarrow and yellow dock.

Supplements: Liquid chlorophyll, lecithin, salmon oil, evening primrose oil, germanium, coenzyme Q_{10}, glucomannan and blue-green algae (enhances oxygen utilization). L-carnitine helps to lower cholesterol and clean the veins and heart.

Avoid: Red meats—all meat at first—because it puts too much stress on veins and is hard to digest. Avoid salt, sugar, white flour products, alcohol, caffeine drinks, cookies, candy and pastries. Avoid a high-fat diet. Fats circulating in the blood begin to adhere to each other and grow. This creates sticky masses of material that are deposited on the vessel walls, become brittle and inhibit blood circulation. This hard material can break off, float around and cause a stroke or heart attack by blocking the flow of blood and oxygen.

❖ Hyperactivity and ADD

Hyperactivity causes major difficulties and frustration in many homes in America. It is commonly seen in children, but I have seen adults that suffer with this problem. I feel that hypoglycemia in adults is an extension of hyperactivity in children. Many adults cannot cope with life's problems and take tranquilizers and drugs that only complicate the problem and cause a frustrating family life. Hyperactivity is so common and puts such a stress on families that it can lead to marital difficulties, divorce and even child abuse. The condition of hyperactivity is now commonly linked with attention deficit disorder (ADD).

A high percentage of hyperactive children grow up to be troubled teenagers who are involved in drugs, dropping out, crimes, depression, etc. A poor diet is usually a common thread in all problem cases. Seventy-five percent of criminals were hyperactive children and more than half have abnormal glucose tolerance tests. It would appear that diet, hyperactivity and hypoglycemia are often connected to criminal behavior. Hyperactivity and other disorders may result from allergies, created by bad eating habits and nutritional deficiencies. Too much sugar leaches nutrients from the body.

Some of the symptoms of hyperactivity are that a child squirms and fidgets, cannot sit still very long, has a short attention span, and runs instead of walks. The child is into everything, talks constantly in a loud voice, has trouble following instructions, and is often moody. A hyperactive child is often impulsive, and forgets easily.

Ritalin is widely prescribed for hyperactive children—it is being used on more than a million children. But this drug is not the answer. Dr. Robert Mendelsohn says, "Educators who don't like unruly pupils have, with the willing help of doctors and psychologists, broadened the definition of hyperactivity to include a substantial percentage of those in the country who are under age twenty-one. As a consequence, for the comfort and convenience of teachers and parents, millions of normally lively kids have been drugged with Ritalin and turned into virtual zombies by its effects."

Natural Therapy: Lower bowel cleansing and blood purifiers. The bowels, when not kept clean and eliminating every day, will accumulate toxins in the blood. The brain and nervous system are very sensitive to these poisons. Keep food colorings, preservatives, sweets from those prone to hyperactivity. Children are very prone to cadmium and lead contamination and a hair analysis will determine whether there is heavy metal poisoning in the body. .

Foods to Heal: Foods high in B-complex vitamins: whole grains (thermos cooking to retain vitamins and enzymes), buckwheat, millet, wheat, cornmeal, barley, and brown rice. Also healing are sunflower seeds, almonds, wild rice, brewer's yeast, molasses, wheat and oat bran, soybeans, egg yolk, sprouts and green leafy vegetables.

Vitamins and Minerals: Vitamin A (protects against allergies), B-complex vitamins with extra B_5, B_6, B_{12} and niacin, vitamin C with bioflavonoids, multiminerals with extra calcium, magnesium, selenium and zinc.

Herbal Combinations: Allergies, bone, glands, immune, lower bowel, nervine, stress.

Single Herbs: Key herbs are black walnut (kills parasites), burdock (cleans blood), catnip (relaxing), dandelion (cleans liver), gotu kola (brain food), hops, lady's slipper (relaxes), lobelia, red clover, skullcap (builds nerves) and wood betony. Other important herbs are alfalfa, chaparral, chickweed, echinacea, goldenseal, yellow dock and yucca.

Supplements: Bee pollen, blue-green algae, rice bran syrup and essential
fatty acids such as salmon oil, evening primrose oil, flaxseed oil (not
rancid), or whole flaxseed soaked in water.

Avoid: All sugar products, white flour products, soft drinks, salt, meat,
hot dogs, lunch meats, preservatives and food colorings. Watch all
food labeling and use only pure foods.

❖ HYPERTHYROIDISM AND HYPOTHYROIDISM

Hyperthyroidism occurs when the thyroid gland produces too much
thyroxine hormone, resulting in an overactive metabolism. Symptoms of
hyperthyroidism are: irritability, weakness, intolerance, rapid heartbeat,
fatigue, insomnia, sweating, etc.

When the thyroid gland produces too little thyroxine hormone, the
condition is known as hypothyroidism. Symptoms of hypothyroidism
are (and the symptoms are frequently missed because they can be associated with other diseases): muscle cramps, low back pain, anemia, easy
bruising, fatigue, PMS, hair loss, muscle weakness, recurrent infections,
depression, and, on occasion, a cold feeling.

It is possible to correct unbalanced thyroid hormone production,
whether it be too much or too little, by correcting vitamin and mineral
deficiencies. All glands are involved when one gland is in trouble.
Essential fatty acids deficiency causes an unbalanced thyroid, so evening
primrose oil has helped many people with this disease. Any essential
fatty acid will improve symptoms. Shortage of vitamins C and E can
bring on hyperthyroidism, so supplements can help alleviate the problem.

Dr. Broda O. Barnes, M.D. developed a self-test to determine the
severity of hypothyroidism: take a thermometer and shake it down and
put it on your bedstand. Immediately upon awakening in the morning,
place the thermometer snugly in the armpit for ten minutes by the
clock. A reading below the normal range of 97.8 to 98.2 strongly suggests low thyroid function. If the reading is above the normal range, one
must be suspicious of some infection or an overactive thyroid gland.

Natural Therapy: Blood purifiers, lymphatic cleansing and lower bowel
cleansers. Raw foods are necessary for the glandular system. Cooking

❖

food kills enzymes and causes the endocrine glands to become over-worked, leading to body autoxidation and causing diseases such as hypothyroidism and hyperthyroidism. Cooked foods overstimulate the gland and cause the body to retain excess weight. The enzymes from live food help the body to maintain proper metabolism. Problems arise when the glands do not receive the nutrients necessary to satisfy the body's needs. When this happens, the glands overstim-ulate the digestive organs and demand more food. This produces an oversecretion of hormones and an unhealthy appetite, which finally results in exhaustion of the hormone-producing glands.

Foods to Heal: Live foods, sprouts, salads, raw fruit and vegetables are excellent. Eat grains and rice that are thermos-cooked to retain the enzymes which heal and feed the glands. Seeds and nuts, such as sesame seeds, pumpkin seeds, sunflower seeds, almonds, pecans and cashews (raw and unsalted) are nourishing to the glands. Raw veg-etable juices (carrot, celery, parsley, comfrey) and green drinks con-tain chlorophyll for a healthy blood. Seaweeds are another healing food.

Vitamins and Minerals: Vitamin A assists in maintaining normal glan-dular function. B-complex vitamins are necessary to help control glandular health. They build the adrenals, thyroid and calm the nerves. Vitamin C promotes normal adrenal function and glandular activity. A deficiency is seen in thyroid problems.Vitamins D and E work together with vitamin A. Vitamin E is essential for glandular health—it protects the B vitamins from rapid oxidation. Vitamin F, found in essential fatty acids, is a must for glandular health. It improves overall health. All minerals are involved in glandular health. Calcium and magnesium support the glands and manganese, seleni-um, silicon and zinc protect the glands.

Herbal Combinations: Blood purifiers, bone, digestion, glands, immune, nervine, stress.

Single Herbs: For the adrenals use: licorice (stimulates the glands), rose hips (rich in vitamin C and B-vitamins), capsicum and ginseng (strengthens the body). For the pituitary: alfalfa, licorice, ginseng, gotu kola and ho-shou-wu. For the thyroid: black walnut, kelp, white oak bark. For the female glands: black cohosh, dong quai, damiana and yellow dock. For the male glands, use ginseng, kelp and damiana. Other vital herbs are bayberry, blue cohosh, burdock, chaparral, dandelion, garlic, ginger, hawthorn, hops, kelp, lobelia, mistletoe, parsley, sarsaparilla (stimulates glandular function), skullcap, valerian, wood betony and yellow dock.

Supplements: Evening primrose oil, linseed oil, bentonite cleanse, goldenseal and echinacea.

Avoid: All junk food. It overstimulates the glands and causes exhaustion and weakness. Eliminate sugar and white flour products. Fried foods are hard to digest and cause free radicals to form and destroy the cells. Avoid all drugs including the pill, antibiotics, sulfa drugs and tranquilizers. They will put a burden on the glands and cause dysfunction.

✢ HYPOGLYCEMIA

Hypoglycemia means low blood sugar. *Hypo* means "low" and *glycemia* means "sugar". Moods swing drastically, from happy and energetic to anxious, irritable, tearful and depressed. Mental confusion and phobias can also manifest themselves when hypoglycemia is present. Because of the ups and downs in blood sugar that come with hypoglycemia, there is a wear-and-tear on the body that affects the nervous system, the muscles and cells, and the glands. Hypoglycemia is seen as the first step on the road to chronic degenerative disease because of its devastating effect on the body, especially in the stress-related adrenals.

The symptoms of hypoglycemia are very subtle. I have observed many people with hypoglycemia and their actions become so normal to them that they do not realize they are acting in a negative or unusual way. The way they perceive and react to situations becomes distorted.

One friend of mine went through a very traumatic period in her life. She knew that if she divorced her husband all her problems would be solved. Later when she was able to get her hypoglycemia under control, she realized her problems weren't caused by her husband. It was her hypoglycemic condition. Common symptoms of hypoglycemia are anxiety, antisocial behavior, confusion, depression, emotional instability, exhaustion, headaches, impatience, inability to cope, intense hunger, phobias, sugar craving.

There are several causes of hypoglycemia that stem from a diet high in refined food and excessive sugar intake. Stress, glandular dysfunction and mineral deficiencies are also factors. The typical American diet is high in processed food, food chemically treated, overcooked, stripped of nutrients, sweetened, salted and altered in many ways. Fried foods are found in a typical diet and disrupt the glandular system.

Sugar is added to food products to increase consumption. Sugar is a very addictive substance; the low blood sugar you get from eating it makes you crave more. The food industry has discovered that increasing the sugar in a product also increases the amount a person will eat, which will increase sales. White sugar is not a food; it is a chemical which wears out the glandular system.

Many people with hypoglycemia accept it as their fate because it seems to run in their family. But Dr. Robert Atkins, one of the foremost pioneers in the field of blood sugar disturbances, does not agree. He said, "Without improper nutrition, I don't believe diabetes could develop, even if both parents are diabetic. No one is doomed by heredity to develop diabetes, I also feel that we are not doomed to develop hypoglycemia or many of the diseases plagued by mankind, just because our parents have it."

Natural Therapy: Glandular therapy using herbs to strengthen and cleanse the glands. Frequent meals consisting of wholesome food. Since fasting is hard on hypoglycemia, use cleansing drinks and lower bowel formulas to help clean the cells, colon and liver. Parsley, wheat grass, carrot and celery juices and green vegetables build the blood. Chiropractic or reflexology treatments are excellent to help control hypoglycemia along with diet, herbs, vitamins and minerals. Also helpful are stress management and exercise.

Foods to Heal: Sprouts will heal the glands; alfalfa, radish, mung beans, buckwheat, and fenugreek are excellent. Eat a variety of nourishing foods—steamed and fresh vegetables, fresh fruit, fish, chicken (organically grown), rice, baked potatoes, thermos cooked grain and soups.

Vitamins and Minerals: Vitamin A is healing for the glands. B-complex is a must (with extra B_1, B_3, B_5, B_6, B_{12}, pantothenic acid), vitamin C with bioflavonoids, and vitamin E. Multiminerals are essential for

❖

glandular healing. Calcium, magnesium potassium, phosphorus, manganese, iodine, chromium and zinc are also necessary.

Herbal Combinations: Allergies, bone, digestion, endurance, glands, hypoglycemia formulas, immune, nerves.

Single Herbs: Alfalfa (nourishes the glands), black cohosh, cayenne (aids in the circulation of blood so that oxygen and other nutrients reach cells in need of repair), dandelion, garlic, ginger (stimulates blood and cleans capillaries), gotu kola (stimulates the brain and relieves fatigue), hawthorn (strengthens the heart when under stress), juniper berries, kelp (cleans and nourishes the glands), lady's slipper, licorice (feeds the adrenals and provides energy), lobelia, mullein, parsley, saffron (helps digest oils), skullcap and uva ursi.

Supplements: Bee pollen, chlorophyll, green drinks, royal jelly, lecithin, spirulina, wheat grass juice and essential fatty acids.

Avoid: All sugar products, even fruit juices (too concentrated). Small amounts of fruit can be eaten because they are cleansing to the body. Avoid all unnatural food—fried, canned, or overcooked. Eliminate alcohol, tobacco, too much protein and fat, and stimulating foods.

❖ IMMUNE SYSTEM

Our immune system is in great danger from the widespread use of drugs. Tranquilizers, antibiotics and vaccinations are creating so-called "immune-related diseases." According to Dr. Robert Mendelsohn, "There is a growing suspicion that immunization against relatively harmless childhood disease may be responsible for the dramatic increase in autoimmune disease since mass inoculations were introduced."

The key to prevention and treatment of diseases is a healthy, well-functioning immune system. The immune system is genetically-programmed to shelter you from disease. It will protect you if you keep it in top shape. The immune system is equipped with glands, cells, organs, and proteins to fight off autoimmune diseases. With all of the diseases in the world ready to invade the body, the immune system must be prepared to battle these scourges. The body can be weakened to the point that it does not respond to the normal intake of nutrients. The immune system accumulates damage, becomes defective and, consequently, cannot do its job. This problem plays a role in most degenerative diseases.

❖

Immune Related Diseases

AIDS: A devastating disease that alters the body's ability to protect itself by causing a complete breakdown of the immune system. The disease is now reaching epidemic proportions. The AIDS virus, along with over forty other viruses, is found in the kidney of the African green monkey, of which vaccinations are made.

ANKYLOSING SPONDYLITIS: A progressive, inflammatory arthritis characterized by fusion of various joints, especially of the spine.

BACTEREMIA: Occurs when bacteria invade the blood. Bacteremia can result from any infection—an abscess, an inflamed urinary tract, infected female organs, lung infections, intravenous drug use, urinary catheters, surgical procedures, or from any bacteria which get into the blood. When the blood is impure, it creates infection anywhere.

CANCER: A breakdown in the body's immune system. Bad eating habits, impure blood and constipation can cause autointoxication where the toxins circulate in the bloodstream and invade the weakest part of the body.

CANDIDA ALBICANS: A yeast invader that weakens the immune system. It occurs in epidemic proportions and can produce mild symptoms or create pain, fatigue, and mental anguish. Doctors who once freely prescribed antibiotics are now realizing that antibiotics should not be given commonly, as they contribute to infections such as candida. But antibiotics are still given to animals in their feed, assuring a constant supply of them in our food.

CHLAMYDIAL DISEASE: A common sexually transmitted disease that is very serious because it can cause infertility in women, or constant urinary tract and prostatic infection in men.

CRIB DEATH (SUDDEN INFANT DEATH SYNDROME): Each year thousands of babies between the ages of four weeks and seven months die in their sleep. Crib death may result from a breakdown in a child's immune systems. Babies are born with naturally low immunity, but acquire a certain amount from the mothers' antibodies in the placenta. SIDS is preponderantly a disease thay affects artificially fed infants. Bottle-fed babies suffer from deficiencies in oxygen. This causes bacteria to become pathogenic, parasitic and virulent. Virulent bacteria produces viruses which exhaust vitamins C and A as well as minerals in the body.

EPSTEIN-BARR VIRUS: This is a disease that is considered a cancer-triggering virus. This virus is found in the kidney of the African green monkey, which is used in vaccinations. This virus was once thought to be harmless but is now known to play a leading role in a deadly and horribly disfiguring cancer that strikes the noses and throats of some fifty thousand people a year. It has also been associated with an immune cell cancer (Burkitt's lymphoma) that is usually found in children.

GASTRITIS: This is a superficial inflammation of the stomach lining. It is caused by drugs, stress, alcohol, and by toxins recirculating in our blood because of autointoxication. Aspirin, cortisone, antibiotics and nonprescription drugs can wear away at our stomach lining. Gastritis can become chronic and cause serious problems such as ulcers or cancer if it is not taken care of.

LEGIONNAIRE'S DISEASE: This disease is caused by a breakdown in the immune system. It occurs more often in persons who are middle-aged or elderly and who have lymphoma or other disorders. It receives its name from the peculiar, highly publicized illness that struck 182 people (29 of whom died) at an American Legion convention in Philadelphia the summer of 1976. It is an acute bronchopneumonia produced by a gram-negative bacillus. (The bacillus was found in the air conditioning in the building where the meeting was held.) Again, the immune system plays a vital role in protecting us from this sickness.

LUPUS ERYTHEMATOSUS: A systemic autoimmune disease that usually strikes young women. It is a connective tissue disease that causes inflammation. A second type of lupus, discoid lupus, is much less serious, affecting only the skin. But both kinds need nutrients and a healthy diet to keep them under control.

REYE'S SYNDROME: This is a childhood disease that targets children under eighteen. Parents have been warned not to give their children aspirin if they are suspected of having chicken pox or the flu. This combination seems to precipitate the syndrome. The disease produces fever, vomiting and disturbances of consciousness, progressing to coma and convulsions. It causes fatty infiltration of the liver and kidneys, with cerebral edema and many other destructive effects. A weakened immune system promotes susceptibility to this disease.

❖

TOXIC SHOCK SYNDROME: This disease affects menstruating women in their late teens or early twenties. It afflicts those who use highly absorbent synthetic fiber tampons, thought to trigger *Staphylococcus aureus.* This organism produces the toxins that cause toxic shock syndrome. One cause of TSS could be the lack of magnesium. Many women have been stricken by this disease quite suddenly. In 1985 it was reported that 114 women died from this disease. These women usually experienced nausea, diarrhea, and dizziness, accompanied by a sudden high fever. This was often followed by a rash, peeling skin, and possibly shock, unconsciousness and paralysis. A sharp drop in blood pressure is another symptom of this syndrome. Recovery is often a long and painful process.

Natural Therapy: Blood purifiers, lower bowel cleaners, nervine therapies to keep the immune system strong. The nervous system is connected to the immune system and when one is weakened the other one becomes weak. Change to a healthy diet because all nutrients positively affect the immune system. Exercise often. Do not let stressful situations control how you act. Fresh, clean air is vital for the lungs and immune system.

Foods to Heal: Fish, vegetables such as broccoli, cabbage, cauliflower, brussels sprouts, parsley, chicken, apples, apricots, bananas, green beans, berries, cherries, corn, leaf lettuce (lots of salads), melons, okra, peaches, fresh peas, potatoes, prunes, plums, watercress, sprouts, brown rice, millet, buckwheat, pineapple, yellow cornmeal, rye, goat's milk.

Vitamins and Minerals: Vitamins A, E, and C are important for many reasons, especially for their antioxidant qualities that protect the immune system. Vitamin A increases resistance to infections and protects against pollution, cancer and viral infections. Vitamin E prevents the oxidized state in which cancer cells thrive. It deactivates free radicals that promote cellular damage and lead to malignancy. Vitamin C can activate white blood cells to battle foreign substances and increase the production of interferon, the body's antivirus protein. B-complex vitamins are also vital—they protect the nervous system, prevent fatigue, and increase resistance to disease.

❖

Multiminerals with extra selenium and zinc manifest anti-carcinogenic and anti-mutagenic properties. Selenium inhibits breast, skin, liver, and colon cancer. It is lost in food processing. Zinc is vital for the immune system. It produces histamine which dilates the capillaries so that blood, carrying immune-fighting white blood cells, can hurry to the scene of an infection. Calcium prevents heavy metals from accumulating in the body; magnesium produces properdin, a blood protein that fights invading viruses and bacteria; and manganese activates enzymes that work with vitamin C. Also use iodine, iron and chromium.

Herbal Combinations: Blood purifiers, bone, candida, digestion, glands, immune formulas, lower bowels, nerves.

Single Herbs: All herbs are good for the immune system. Key herbs are burdock (blood cleanser), ginkgo (helps in circulation), ginseng (strengthens the whole body), goldenseal (a great cleanser and healer), capsicum (cleans the veins), chaparral (cell cleanser), echinacea (lymphatic and blood cleanser), garlic (antibiotic properties), kelp, lobelia, mullein, pau d'arco, red clover, suma and watercress.

Supplements: Acidophilus, bee pollen, blue-green algae, and essential fatty acids are vital to overall health.

Avoid: Alcohol, tobacco, drugs of all kinds, tranquilizers, all sugar products, and white flour products. They have no food value and deplete vital nutrients.

❖ IMPOTENCE

Impotence is the inability to achieve or maintain an erection. In can develop because of mental and physical fatigue and stress. Tension will create the inability to perform sexually by reducing blood flow to vessels of the penis. Anxiety, fatigue, depression, unhappiness, marital problems, anger, hate and a poor self-image can contribute to impotence.

Antidepressants, tranquilizers, antihypertensive drugs, and antiulcer drugs are some examples of medications which can cause impotence.

I believe that nutritional deficiency and autointoxication are two very real causes of this problem. Proper circulation without cholesterol buildup in the veins is important. A positive mental outlook can be achieved when good health habits are implemented.

❖

Natural Therapy: Blood purifying, building up the nerves, and lower bowel cleansing to eliminate toxic buildup in the body. Exercise to help with blood circulation and build a healthy heart. Try to achieve a good self-image through a proper attitude. Create love, happiness and joy through nutrition and a healthy mental outlook.

Foods to Heal: Fruit is important because it cleanses the body. Apples, oranges, lemons, grapefruit, bananas, papaya, grapes, cherries and all kinds of berries, peaches, pears and apricots are good. Whole grains contain essential minerals such as zinc, selenium, manganese, copper, chromium, all necessary for a healthy sex life. Sprouts contain live enzymes. Seeds are important because they can create living food and therefore are good for the body. Beans, lentils, and peas are all good food.

Vitamins and Minerals: Lack of vitamin A will cause sterility and loss of vitality and vigor. It is essential for a healthy and strong body. B-complex vitamins (with extra B_3, B_4, B_6, B_{12}, folic acid and PABA) prevent nervous disorders, are nutritional stimulants, utilize energy in the brain and nervous system and protect against stress. Vitamin C with bioflavonoids, vital for all-around health, prevents cholesterol from building up in the veins and protects against stress. It is vital for immune function and protect against viruses and germs. Vitamin E is called the "fertility vitamin." It is essential for the reproductive organs of the male and female. It strengthens the heart muscles and dilates capillary blood vessels, enabling blood to flow more freely into muscle tissue. Multiminerals, selenium and zinc are important. Zinc has a beneficial effect on the prostate and all the glands. It also assists the body in absorbing B-complex vitamins.

Herbal Combinations: Blood purifier, bone (rich in minerals), digestion, energy and fitness formulas, glands, immune, lower bowels and stress formulas.

Single Herbs: Key herbs are damiana (tonic to glands), ginseng (strengthens the body), gotu kola (brain food), ho-shou-wu, kelp, sarsaparilla, saw palmetto, alfalfa, blessed thistle, cramp bark, echinacea, false unicorn and goldenseal.

Supplements: Amino acids, bee pollen, lecithin, chlorophyll and essential fatty acids (salmon oil, evening primrose oil, etc.).

❖

Avoid: Avoid hot baths and saunas which could lead to low sperm counts. Avoid smoking, alcohol, caffeine drinks. Sugar products and white flour products leach nutrients from body. Heavy metal poisoning may lead to energy loss. (Hair analysis can determine a buildup of metals.)

❖ INDIGESTION (DYSPEPSIA)

Indigestion is one of the most common health problems people are faced with today. If you lack hydrochloric acid and enzymes you may have bad breath, heartburn, belching and flatulence. Other problems associated with incomplete digestion are: skin problems, recurring headaches, muscle wasting, lowered immunity, delayed wound healing, anemia, poor bowel function, depression and allergies. If the food stays longer in the digestive tract than it should, constipation and diarrhea and autointoxication develops. Poor digestion is the beginning of many chronic diseases. Digestive disorders are: constipation, diarrhea, acidosis and alkalosis, gastric catarrh, chronic gastritis, dilation of the stomach, ulcers, liver disorders, gallstones, enteritis, appendicitis, colitis, diverticulosis and hemorrhoids.

The stomach is the most abused organ of the body. Americans treat themselves with antacids, which are swallowed in unbelievable amounts each year. Along with tranquilizers and sleeping pills, antacids are the most commonly prescribed drug used today. But antacids are not the answer. Although they offer initial relief, the stomach reacts by producing even more acid because the cause of an acid stomach has not been dealt with. Antacids slow down digestion and create flatulence. Many people use bicarbonate of soda, but it is high in salt and constant use can cause kidney stones. It also produces carbon dioxide in the stomach, resulting in belching and distension.

Hydrochloric acid is necessary for digestion and good health. It is essential for the assimilation and absorption of minerals and vitamins because this process begins in the stomach. Hydrochloric acid also destroys many harmful bacteria, parasites, and worms that could enter the bloodstream and be carried to other parts of the body. If the bacteria, parasites and worms are not destroyed, they can set up colonies in the intestine and interfere with the absorption of food nutrients.

❖

Natural Therapy: Blood purification, liver cleansers and a cleansing of the entire gastrointestinal system. Juice fasts along with enemas or lower bowel cleansers are helpful. Healing and cleansing herbs remove obstructions in the colon, stomach, liver and gallbladder. Eat only when you are hungry, avoid large meals, chew food thoroughly with mouth closed (prevents swallowing air). Don't drink liquids with meals because it dilutes the hydrochloric acid.

Foods to Heal: Sprouts, especially alfalfa and fenugreek, provide minerals and cleansing properties. Citrus juice in warm water is healing and cleansing for the digestive tissues. Combining food properly will heal and improve digestion. Don't mix proteins and starches at the same meal. A protein works well with vegetables. Starch meals work well with vegetables. Fiber-rich foods will promote proper digestion. Whole grains, fresh fruits and vegetables, fresh papayas, pineapples and mangos are good digestive aids and provide digestive-enzymes.

Vitamins and Minerals: Vitamin A, along with pantothenic acid and zinc, work together to aid the absorption of nutrients in the intestinal tract. B_{12} needs hydrochloric acid for absorption. A deficiency can cause learning disabilities, nervousness and depression. B-complex vitamins with extra B_1, B_2, B_6, niacinamide and choline are beneficial. Vitamin C with bioflavonoids requires hydrochloric acid for efficient absorption. Minerals are essential for a healthy body and manganese, calcium and other minerals need proper digestion for the body to utilize nutrients.

Herbal Combinations: Blood purifier, bone formulas, digestion, immune, lower bowel, nerve, stress.

Single Herbs: Key herbs are bitter herbs such as gentian and Oregon grape. For a nervous stomach take chamomile tea with ginger. For acid stomach or heartburn take raspberry tea or one tablespoon of slippery elm and a capsule of ginger in warm water. For nausea mix together cinnamon, cardamon, nutmeg, cloves, and a pinch of ginger in a warm cup of herbal tea. Aloe vera juice is healing. Buchu and capsicum promote circulation. Comfrey is healing and will rebuild tissue. Fennel is soothing and garlic, goldenseal and gentian are great healers of the intestinal tract. Ginger, marshmallow (reduces inflammation), papaya, parsley, peppermint, slippery elm, and psyllium are

❖

also healing. Nervine herbs are hops, passionflower, saffron (helps to digest fats), skullcap, and valerian.

Supplements: Bee pollen, acidophilus, aloe vera juice, glucomannan, calcium combination, garlic and peppermint oil. Also use a protein digestive aid and pancreatic enzymes.

Avoid: Antacids and alcohol. Mineral oil blocks vitamins A and B vitamins from being absorbed. Wrong food combining is detrimental, as is eating when upset or under stress. Eliminate excessive salt, sugar, spices, meat, and dairy products. Chew your food well—it has a profound effect on digestion. Avoid white rice, white bread and white sugar; they stimulate production of hydrochloric acid but cannot neutralize them. Coffee speeds up acid production. Stress inhibits gastric secretions. Antibiotics kill the bacteria flora in colon, causing a deficiency of vitamins K and B.

❖ INFERTILITY

After a girl reaches puberty, now around the age of eleven or twelve (it used to be around age sixteen fifty years ago), one egg is released each month until menopause. If the egg is not fertilized by male sperm, the egg is eliminated out of the body and a new one is replaced the next month. With infertility something is usually wrong to either the female egg or the male sperm.

Since infertility is increasing, many American couples experience unhappiness and frustration. It is now known that it is not necessarily the woman's fault, as it was thought in the past. Men are to blame in about 40 percent of the cases. Women's problems are many, and usually include infections, venereal disease, inherited disorders, mishandled abortions, bacterial organisms, endometriosis, drugs, plugged fallopian tubes, emotional trauma or nutritional deficiencies.

Birth control pills were developed about thirty years ago, and women who have used the pill have usually done so without fear, convinced that it was safe and harmless. But the manufacturers of the pill are faced with hundreds of lawsuits a year women suffering from numerous side effects. The pill can cause permanent infertility, high blood pressure, blood clots, strokes, heart disease, kidney failure, varicose veins, and cancer of the breast, uterus and liver.

Natural Therapy: Blood purification, lower bowel cleansing using enemas, colonics or herbal colon cleansers. Autointoxication could be a problem. Change the diet to natural, wholesome food. Sprouts and seeds have life-giving properties, as do nuts, fresh salads, cabbage, and other raw vegetables. Wheat grass juice is an excellent food to build and clean the blood.

Foods to Heal: Fresh raw fruit first thing in the morning. Half a lemon in warm water is a liver booster. Soak whole grains the night before and eat for breakfast. Make almond milk for cereal. Carrot and beet juices are nourishing. Steamed vegetables, sprouts, alfalfa, mung beans, wheat, fenugreek and radish are healthful. Eat lots of fresh fruit and berries in the season. Fish and organic chicken and eggs are nourishing.

Vitamins and Minerals: Vitamin A assists in maintaining normal glandular activity and prevents sterility. B-complex vitamins protect against stress, nausea, edema and toxemia, and stabilize female hormone levels, which is critical in conceiving. Vitamin C and bioflavonoids strengthen male sperm and female eggs and protect against germs and viruses. Lack of this nutrient can cause varicose veins, slow healing of wounds and frequent sickness. Vitamin E is called the fertility vitamin for the male as well as the female. Lack of this vitamin is the major cause of premature babies. Vitamin D is essential in pregnancy to prevent rickets in infants. Multimineral supplementation is also essential. Extra selenium, silicon, calcium, magnesium, manganese, and zinc are critical for conceiving. Kelp is high in iodine, oatstraw is rich in silicon, and an herbal calcium formula is easily assimilated.

Herbal Combinations: Anemia, blood purifier, bone formulas, candida, digestion, female herbal formula, glands, immune, lower bowels, nerve formulas.

Single Herbs: Alfalfa, chickweed, damiana (strengthens reproductive organs), dandelion, dong quai (good for female organs), echinacea (cleans blood), false unicorn (helps in infertility), ginseng (men), kelp, licorice, oatstraw, pau d'arco, red clover, red raspberry (strengthens all female organs), sarsaparilla (stimulates progesterone) and saw palmetto.

Supplements: Acidophilus, chlorophyll, essential fatty acids, evening primrose oil, safflower oil, salmon oil.

Avoid: Drugs of all kinds, even aspirin, can cause birth defects. Avoid all white flour and white sugar. Avoid chlorinated water, chemicals, pesticides, herbicides and heavy metal poisoning. Check mercury and other metal poisoning in the teeth.

❖ INSOMNIA

Insomnia is a major problem in our society today. Many have trouble falling asleep, or they suddenly wake up in the middle of the night and cannot go back to sleep. There are many reasons for insomnia. It could be caused by anxiety, stress, lack of nutrients (especially minerals), hypoglycemia, nervous tension, physical aches and pains, eating heavy meals late at night, or stimulation from cola drinks, coffee, tea and chocolate.

Insomnia is a nervous disorder, and almost all nervous disorders are affected by autointoxication—self-poisoning by chronic constipation. (Remember, no one thinks they are constipated, but because of our eating habits, we do not completely eliminate excess food). The brain and the nervous system are very sensitive to toxins, and when the bloodstream isn't clean and pure, it has a negative effect on sleep.

Prescription drugs for insomnia are not the answer; instead of curing sleeplessness, they only cover the symptoms. Millions of prescription drugs are written each year for sleeping pills and are responsible for thousands of trips to hospital emergency rooms. Many of those victims fail to leave the hospital alive.

Research shows that people with chronic insomnia almost always have nutritional deficiencies. They usually lack B-complex vitamins, vitamin C, vitamin D, calcium, magnesium, manganese, potassium and zinc. These natural nutrients enable our sleep mechanism to function properly. We know that a lack of any B-vitamins can contribute to anxiety, depression and insomnia. If a person wakes up in the morning tired and exhausted it usually means the liver needs purifying and cleansing.

Natural Therapy: Bowel cleanses using enemas, colonics or lower bowel cleansers and a diet to build up the bowels. Nervine therapy to build and strengthen the nerves. Fresh clean air will help induce natural sleep. Relaxation with natural mental therapies. Sleep in cotton garments if possible; the skin is eliminating toxins constantly and this will help skin detoxification.

Foods to Heal: Whole grains, oats, millet (high in magnesium), buckwheat, wheat and barley contain B-complex vitamins. Nuts, seeds (sesame, sunflower, pumpkin), almonds (high in calcium and magnesium). Green vegetables (high in calcium). Sprouts (alfalfa, mung beans, radish, fenugreek). Kale leaves, turnip greens, mustard, spinach.

Vitamins and Minerals: Multivitamins and extra B-complex build the nerves. Vitamin C with bioflavonoids is cleansing, and protects the nerves. Take a multimineral with extra calcium and magnesium (herbal calcium formulas are rich in calcium and minerals). Silicon, manganese, selenium and zinc are also needed.

Herbal Combinations: Blood Purifier, bone, digestion, glands, insomnia formulas, lower bowels, stress.

Single Herbs: Catnip, chamomile (tea), hops (settles the brain), lady's slipper (extract), lobelia (relaxer), passionflower (settles nerves), skullcap (feeds the nerves), valerian (helps in insomnia) and wood betony.

Supplements: Chlorophyll, lecithin and blue-green algae.

Avoid: Coffee, caffeine drinks, drugs, sleeping pills (weakens the nerves), alcohol, junk food.

✤ LUPUS

Lupus is a chronic inflammatory disorder of the connective tissue. It appears in two forms: discoid lupus erythematosus (DLE), which affects only the skin; and systemic lupus erythematosus (SLE), which generally affects other organs as well as the skin. It can be fatal and is characterized by remissions and flareups like its cousin disease rheumatoid arthritis.

There are three theories as to the cause of SLE: First, SLE is an abnormal reaction of the body to its own tissues, caused by a breakdown in the autoimmune system; second, certain factors may make a person more susceptible to SLE than others, such as stress, streptococcal or viral infections, exposure to sunlight, immunization, pregnancy or genetic

❖

predisposition; third, SLE may be aggravated by certain drugs, from anticonvulsants to penicillins, sulfa drugs and oral contraceptives.

Symptoms include non-deforming arthritis (joint pain and stiffness), a "butterfly rash," and sensitivity to light. General body symptoms of SLE may include aching, malaise, fatigue, low-grade fevers, chills, anorexia and arid weight loss. Lymph node enlargement, abdominal pain, nausea, vomiting, diarrhea and constipation may also occur. Heart and kidney problems may occur, and headaches, irritability and depression are also common.

Corticosteroids are the main medical treatment for SLE. But there are no miracle drugs because it is a complex disease. Those who use natural methods of cure have been known to be able to stop using cortisone and other drugs within six months to a year. Lupus, as well as rheumatoid arthritis, is a condition difficult to move out of the body. (Medical doctors and researchers believe that the degenerative diseases we are increasingly suffering from are side effects from the many immunizations people have been given over the past few decades. These immunizations have the effect of making it impossible for our immune systems to know whether a substance in the body is its own or whether it comes from the outside the body.)

Herbs, diet, and other therapies that would normally help move out toxic waste matter and mucus with other ailments, do not treat SLE. The waste simply stirs around in the bloodstream, unable to be removed from the body. This is because the body's ability to remove accumulated waste is hindered and retarded by a constant buildup of parasites. When the parasites are killed, nature has a better chance to cleanse.

Another cause is that protein molecules from dairy products (pasteurized and homogenized) can readily pass through the intestinal wall and form antigen antibody complexes which can cause arthritis and form the complexes of SLE.

Natural Therapy: Use blood purifiers with herbs that destroy worms and parasites. Cleansing the bowels and the liver needs to be considered. A change of diet is the first consideration. Large amounts of naturally cleansing foods like raw vegetable and fruit juices, as well as a mild food diet, are the only ways to heal this disease. A fast of water and

❖

juices could also be used to great effect, as well as garlic, catnip and cayenne enemas. Mild to moderate exercise will help. Massage of the extremities and central nervous system at regular intervals would give the body a great deal of extra support in moving toxins out. Systemic lupus is a degenerative disease whose power and final outcome depend largely upon the mental, physical, emotional and spiritual attitude of the sufferer. Never give up—the nature of a degenerative disease is that the body is in an unnatural and confused state.

Foods to Heal: Endive, whole oats, lentils, beans, split peas, whole wheat, barley, brown rice, asparagus, green peas and sunflower seeds. Green salads (using leaf lettuce only) with lemon and olive oil dressing. Broccoli, cabbage, brussels sprouts, almonds, avocados, buckwheat, millet, salmon, chickpeas, parsley and watercress.

Vitamins and Minerals: Vitamin A builds up the immune system, B-complex with PABA is needed, vitamin C with bioflavonoids is essential for the connective tissues, and vitamins E and D also help. Multiminerals, especially manganese, magnesium, calcium and the trace minerals, silicon, selenium and zinc, are essential for all healing.

Herbal Combinations: Arthritis, blood purifier, bone, chelation formulas, digestion, immune, lower bowels, nerve, potassium.

Single Herbs: The nervine herbs should be considered first. They are: black cohosh, hops, lobelia, passionflower, skullcap, valerian and willow bark. Black walnut and goldenseal will kill parasites and worms. Garlic and chaparral are excellent cleansers. Other important herbs are aloe vera, burdock (blood cleanser), capsicum, comfrey (healing to the skin and mucous membranes), dandelion (helps the liver to detoxify), devil's claw (cleans deep in the cells), echinacea (cleans blood and lymphatics), eyebright, fenugreek, ginger, hawthorn, licorice, lobelia, myrrh, oatstraw, Oregon grape, pau d'arco (blood purifier), red clover (cleans toxins from the blood), white oak, yellow dock, yucca and watercress.

Supplements: Acidophilus, carrot and celery juice, chelated cell salts, Chinese essential oils (use externally for pain), evening primrose oil, fish oil lipids, salmon oil, germanium and coenzyme Q_{10}.

Avoid: All white sugar and white flour products. Eliminate meat, fried food, stimulants such as alcohol, caffeine, tobacco, and all other

❖

drugs. Avoid sunlight. Avoid birth control pills and antibiotics. Avoid too much salt.

❖ MENIERE'S SYNDROME (RINGING IN EARS, TINNITUS)

The hearing nerve is closely connected with the nerve leading from the balancing mechanism located in the innermost portion of the ear. Disturbances of the balancing mechanism may cause so much ringing in the ears that it can cause hearing impairment. Meniere's syndrome has many symptoms which can affect both ears. Ringing in the ears, loss of hearing, and loss of balance are the most common. Because of balance problems nausea and vomiting may occur. Acute attacks can be so severe that one may actually keel over from the violent dizziness.

A bad diet causes plugged up ears. Mucus-forming foods can cause an accumulation of material in the head area and especially the ears. The head area requires more nutrition and circulation than any other single body organ. Poor nutrition causes tiny arteries, veins, and capillaries that help support ears and hearing to clog up. This happens over a period of years with gradual clogging up of the tubes to the ears. That is why we see so many elderly people with hearing problems. But it is not only the elderly who are having hearing problems; we are seeing more and more children and even newborns with hearing problems. A factor causing hearing loss in our youth is noise pollution. Our ears are not meant to be exposed to loud noises for long periods of time. Nerve damage can result.

Some other causes of hearing loss are fetal damage, trauma at birth, infections, drugs (people have complained of hearing problems after being treated with drugs [quinine is one example]), thyroid disease, diabetes, injuries, noise exposure, or nerve deterioration and malnutrition. We have to realize that a lack of nutrients can contribute to hearing loss.

Natural Therapy: Blood purification, lower bowel cleansing, and toning of digestive organs, nerves and kidneys. Diet change is the most important thing you can do to help change the inward health. Mucus-forming food is the cause of most hearing problems and infections in small children. These infections can build up throughout the

✦

years and cause other ear problems. Herbal tinctures in the ears have helped many people. They help to get circulation in the head area, as well as supplying essential nutrients.

Foods to Heal: Grape juice and green drinks are high in potassium. High potassium prevents autointoxication and a buildup of mucus in the ears. Eat almonds, baked potatoes with skin, apples, apricots (dried), cashews, sunflower seeds, black cherries, broccoli, carrots, dates, dried figs, leaf lettuce, lentils, dried beans and whole grains (thermos cooked). A natural diet is high in whole grains, fresh vegetables, fruits, nuts, seeds, sprouts, legumes, beans.

Vitamins and Minerals: The B-complex vitamins are very important. Extra B_1, B_2, and niacin are vital for balancing the body. Hypoglycemia has been connected with Meniere's syndrome. A multivitamin supplement with extra C and E is required and a multimineral supplement is important. All minerals, especially selenium, manganese, zinc, calcium and magnesium, are crucial. One cause of fluid and pressure imbalance in the inner ear is electrolyte imbalance.

Herbal Combinations: Blood cleanser, hypoglycemia, glands, lower bowels, nerve formulas.

Single Herbs: Key herbs are black cohosh, black walnut (sometimes parasites in the head area can cause hearing problems), burdock, echinacea, garlic (in ears), ginkgo, gotu kola, hawthorn, hops, kelp (high in potassium and other minerals), lady's slipper, licorice, lobelia, red clover (blood purifier) and yellow dock. Other beneficial herbs are buchu, capsicum, chickweed, cornsilk, dandelion, ginger, ginseng, mistletoe, Oregon grape, parsley, queen of the meadow, sarsaparilla, skullcap, St. John's wort, suma, uva ursi, wood betony, yarrow, yucca and watercress.

Supplements: Bee pollen, evening primrose oil, salmon oil, fish oil lipids, blue-green algae.

Avoid: Fried foods, white flour products, and white sugar products. Eliminate smoking, alcohol, caffeine, and a high-meat diet. Exposure to cigarette smoke in the household can cause chronic middle ear disease in children and smoke is dangerous for children who have lung and nasal congestion. Ear damage increases six fold in children that are exposed to secondhand smoke in their formative years.

❖

❖ MENINGITIS

Meningitis is an inflammation of the meninges, the membranes that cover the brain and the spinal cord. It usually occurs in children and is a serious disease that needs to be diagnosed and treated immediately by a medical doctor. It was once a dreaded disease but if treated early with sulfa medicines and antibiotics, it can usually be cured. Mendelsohn cautions that "potential consequences of failure to diagnose and treat meningitis properly are mental retardation and death. If your child has an unexplained fever for three or four days, accompanied by drowsiness, vomiting, a shrill cry, and possibly a stiff neck, it is time to suspect meningitis. Some of these symptoms are also present with influenza. But you can distinguish meningitis by the last two, particularly the shrill cry."

Natural Therapy: Prevention is the best treatment. Blood purification and keeping the bowels open and clean are both therapeutic. Make sure the diet is nutritious and includes a variety of fruits and vegetables. Don't just limit a few vegetables for children, get them acquainted with all good fruit and vegetables. Use brown rice and millet because they digest easily. Use whole grains after a baby is a year old, or has its teeth. The digestion of starches depends on chewing and saliva.

Foods to Heal: Fresh citrus juices made from oranges, lemons, limes and grapefruit are healing. Herbal teas made from catnip, chamomile, peppermint, spearmint, red raspberry, and red clover blends will heal and help the body eliminate toxins. All green vegetables are healing. Use raw finger vegetables for children, including carrots, broccoli, cucumbers, turnips, green peppers, and all raw vegetables. Children need minerals and B-complex vitamins which are found in whole grains. Cook them in a thermos overnight and they will retain their B-vitamins.

Vitamins and Minerals: Vitamins A and C will help the healing process as well as prevent viruses and germs. Take extra B-complex with pantothenic acid. Multiminerals are needed because vomiting and high fevers lead to mineral loss. Zinc is very healing. Calcium and magnesium help protect the nerves.

Herbal Combinations: Blood purifier, bone (rich in minerals), glands, immune, infections formulas, lower bowels, nerves, potassium.

Single Herbs: Key herbs are black walnut (balances minerals), burdock (blood cleanser), capsicum, cascara sagrada (cleans the bowels), catnip (calms the nerves), fenugreek (loosens and eliminates mucus), goldenseal (antiseptic), ginkgo, gotu kola, hops (helps to settle nerves), lady's slipper, lobelia (great nervine and clears obstruction), psyllium (bowel cleanser) and skullcap (helps calm nerves). Other vital herbs are aloe vera, black cohosh, buckthorn, buchu, comfrey, cornsilk, dandelion, hawthorn, horsetail, ho-shou-wu, licorice, myrrh, oatstraw, red clover, rose hips and white oak.

Supplements: Chlorophyll, liquid vitamin C, blue-green algae and lots of liquids. Enemas will help bring a fever down quickly.

Avoid: All white sugar products, artificial sweeteners, flavorings, and colorings. Immunizations have been linked with meningitis. It has to be up to the parents whether to vaccinate their children or not.

✤ MENOPAUSE

Menopause is the physical and emotional transition that marks the permanent cessation of menstruation, and takes approximately five years. It usually starts around the age of fifty. It can take longer if a women is in poor mental and physical health. Symptoms relating to menopause are hot flashes, night sweats, depression, dizziness, headache, difficult breathing, and heart palpitations. These have been connected with a decrease in estrogen production. However, if a women is in good health, has good digestive and eliminative systems, and maintains a positive outlook, these symptoms will hardly be noticed.

With good health habits, the ovaries produce a reduced amount of estrogen following menopause while other glands take over. The adrenals begin to form a type of female hormone which is used along with the small amount of ovarian estrogen. With the right herbs, the body can continue producing the correct amount of hormones needed by the system. Even the correct amount of progesterone is produced by other glands.

Women going through menopause need to decrease the number of calories they eat because their need is less. If they don't, weight gain is more than likely. The body can compensate for the weight gain if complex carbohydrates are added to the diet, in tandem with more vegetables and increased exercise.

Some women start menopause early, some later. Some fertility pills can throw women into menopause way before their time. Drugs can even cause menopausal symptoms. The following drugs can cause cessation of menstruation for varying periods of time, sometimes permanently: oral contraceptives, busulfan, chlorambucil, mechlorethamine, vincristine, and cyclophosphamide.

Natural Therapy: Blood purification, strengthening the glands, and nervine therapy. The liver needs to be strengthened and purified. The liver has the job of filtering toxins to prevent the blood from accumulating excess hormones. Diet change is helpful in cleaning the blood and bowels.

Foods to Heal: Whole grains, sesame and sunflower seeds, almonds, pecans and walnuts are nourishing. Eat lots of vegetables in fresh salads and lightly steamed. Use garlic, figs, dates, cabbage, broccoli, seaweeds, bananas, avocados, grapes. All fruits, fresh and juiced, are healing. Foods rich in magnesium are beans, grains and dark green vegetables.

Vitamins and Minerals: B-complex vitamins will help in nervous disorders, especially B_5 (helps in glandular function), B_6 (helps in water retention), and B_{12} (helps in stressful situations). Vitamin C with bioflavonoids helps with hot flashes. Vitamin E helps in all symptoms of menopause, especially hot flashes. A multivitamin and a multimineral should be taken with meals because they help the body to produce it own hormones. Calcium and magnesium relieve stress and calm the nerves. Selenium is involved in balancing hormones. Silicon, manganese and other trace minerals help the body to utilize calcium.

Herbal Combinations: Anemia (blood building formulas), bone (strengthens the bones and prevents bone loss), digestion formulas (help to assimilate nutrients), glands, nerve and formulas for menopause.

Single Herbs: Key herbs are black cohosh (helps the body make its own hormones), blessed thistle, burdock (blood cleanser), chamomile, damiana (helps to balance hormones), dong quai (great for all female problems), false unicorn, gentian, gotu kola, hawthorn, hops, horsetail (contains silicon for bone health), kelp, red raspberry, sarsaparilla, squaw vine and saw palmetto. Other helpful herbs are alfalfa, licorice, lobelia, parsley, red clover, skullcap (strengthens the nerves), valerian, wood betony and yellow dock.

Supplements: Evening primrose oil, fish oil lipids, salmon oil, chlorophyll, and safflower oil.

Avoid: Dairy products contain antibiotics and hormones to disrupt the body's natural estrogen: milk, cream, cottage cheese, sour cream, cream cheese all contain hormones. Eliminate sugar and white four products. Avoid meat as it can contribute to hot flashes. Avoid coffee, tea, alcohol, nicotine and all drugs—they disrupt the body and cause many side effects.

❖ MENTAL ILLNESS (MANIC-DEPRESSIVE DISORDER, SCHIZOPHRENIA)

Some symptoms of mental disorders are loss of interest in school or work, changes in sleep pattern, withdrawal from society, irritability, panic attacks, sudden attacks of rage, lack of enthusiasm, or loss of interest in family and friends.

I was astonished when a lovely and delightful woman I know, Heather, told me she had been diagnosed as a manic depressive and a borderline schizophrenic. At age thirty she had been hospitalized for a suicide attempt. All her life she had been plagued with mental problems, and her family members had the same problems. She said that desire to commit suicide and panic attacks were a way of life for her. She was on all kinds of drug therapy, including lithium, haldol and oxazepan. She underwent psychiatric therapy two times a week, but nothing seemed to help. Heather's life changed, however, when she was introduced to a nutritional approach to her problem by a friend. With a complete cleansing program and using herbs to clean her blood and colon, she began to gain her sanity. She started out slowly with changes in her diet. She used nervine herbs such as valerian, lady's slipper, passionflower, skullcap, hops, and wood betony. After a time she was able to have her first night of restful sleep in years. She felt her health improve and she

＊

gave up her medications. Her attitude is positive, and she is now well and happy, helping others who suffer from depression.

When someone you know is manifesting symptoms of antisocial behavior, before you make an appointment with a psychiatrist, please examine their diet. Is it loaded with artificial additives, white sugar, donuts, and pastries? Does the person smoke, drink, or consume an inordinate amount of caffeine? Poor nutrition can be a key element in many mental disorders.

Natural Therapy: Blood purification and lower bowel cleansing. Autointoxication is the main cause of mental illness. Toxins can enter the bloodstream and cause all kinds of disturbances. The brain and nervous system are very sensitive to toxins so a change of diet and habits are essential.

Foods to Heal: Whole grains, millet, buckwheat, whole wheat, barley and yellow corn meal (contains vitamin E and B-vitamins). Cold-pressed oils, beans, legumes, brown rice, nuts (almonds, cashew) and seeds. Eat vegetable salads using dark green leafy vegetables. Use steamed vegetables, organic eggs and fish. Fruits have a cleansing effect on the body.

Vitamins and Minerals: A multivitamin with extra vitamins E, A, and C will strengthen the nervous and immune system. B-complex vitamins are necessary for nerves and iron absorption. Vitamin F (essential fatty acids) promotes healing. Take a multimineral with extra calcium, magnesium, silicon, selenium and zinc. Iron (found in yellow dock) is good for energy and oxygen.

Herbal Combinations: Blood purifiers, bone, digestion, lower bowel cleansers, gland formulas, liver formulas, nerves, stress.

Single Herbs: Key herbs are black cohosh, blue vervain, catnip, chamomile, dandelion (liver cleanser), hops, horsetail (supplies silicon and calcium), kelp (rich in minerals), lady's slipper, lobelia, passionflower, psyllium, skullcap and valerian. Other vital herbs are alfalfa, aloe vera, black walnut, buchu, burdock (cleans the blood), capsicum (provides circulation), cascara sagrada, echinacea, garlic, gentian (heals digestive tract), ginger, hawthorn, licorice, parsley, red clover, uva ursi and yellow dock.

Supplements: Essential fatty acids (evening primrose oil, salmon oil, and safflower oil, cold pressed), chlorophyll, lecithin and blue-green algae.

Avoid: Sugar and all sugar-containing food. Eat very little meat; turkey, chicken and fish are best. Eliminate all caffeine products like chocolate and all refined foods.

❖ MONONUCLEOSIS

Mononucleosis is caused by the Epstein-Barr virus, a member of the herpes group. It affects mostly young adults and is rarely seen after age thirty-five. It is an infectious viral disease that affects the lymph tissues and glands in the neck, groin, armpits and in the respiratory system. The symptoms are extreme fatigue, headaches, fever, sore throat, swelling of the glands of the neck and sometimes under the arms and in the groin. It also affects the spleen and the liver.

Mononucleosis is an acute infectious disease that spreads easily. Those with low immune systems who suffer from improper nutrition and exhaustion are the most vulnerable. When mononucleosis is treated naturally, the process will have a positive effect on the body. But if treated with drugs, and if a lot of heavy food is eaten, the disease will embed itself in the system and weaken the organs that are filled with toxins, namely the spleen and the liver.

This disease can be transmitted by blood transfusions and has been reported after cardiac surgery. This is a disease where the virus is in the body, and when it becomes active, the immune system is weakened. It is another disease that could be the result of the mass inocculation that is pushed in our society.

Natural Therapy: Bed rest is essential. Blood purification and lower bowel cleansers are also therapeutic. Strengthen the immune system. Cleanse the body and help nature rid the toxins that are causing the disease. Citrus juices are excellent diluted with fresh pure water. Herbal teas help nature—red clover blend teas and tinctures are excellent. (Read the section on acute diseases to determine how vital it is to treat this disease properly.)

Foods to Heal: Citrus juices at first, then add fresh fruit and vegetables. Eat baked potatoes with the skins on and potassium broths using potato peelings, celery, parsley, chives, onions, cabbage and any vegetable tops. Baked squash is a healing food as are all kinds of vegetables (steamed and fresh). Use only fish, turkey or chicken. Try to get those organically grown to eliminate antibiotics and hormones. Use only whole grains. They contain B-vitamins, minerals and enzymes (if cooked in a thermos overnight).

Vitamins and Minerals: Vitamin A builds the immune system and strengthens the glands. B-complex vitamins help with stress and build up the nerves. Extra B_{12} will help. Vitamin C with bioflavonoids will protect the glands and immune system. It will help the healing process. Vitamin E sends oxygen to the cells and blood. Take a multimineral supplement with extra calcium and magnesium (using herbal calcium formulas). Magnesium helps counter fatigue. Potassium, silicon, selenium and zinc are also beneficial.

Herbal Combinations: Bladder and kidney formulas, blood purifiers, bone, glands, immune and infection formulas.

Single Herbs: Key herbs are burdock, chaparral, dandelion (protects the liver), echinacea (cleans the glands), goldenseal (great for infections), hops, horsetail, lobelia, pau d'arco (cleans the blood and protects the liver) and red clover. Other vital herbs are alfalfa, black walnut, buchu (cleans the kidneys), capsicum, cedar berries, cornsilk, ginger, hawthorn, licorice, parsley, uva ursi, watercress (builds and cleans), yarrow and yellow dock.

Supplements: Acidophilus, liquid chlorophyll, and essential fatty acids such as evening primrose oil, cold-pressed safflower or sunflower seed oil, and salmon oil. Supplement with the amino acid L-lysine. In fact, a free-form amino acid supplement would be helpful. Blue-green algae is also very healing.

Avoid: Chocolate, all sugar products, candy, cake, cookies, ice cream, jams, pastries. Avoid a high meat diet. Eliminate caffeine drinks. All these foods leach nutrients from the body that are essential to a healthy immune and nervous system. Avoid tobacco and alcohol.

✦ MOTION SICKNESS

Motion sickness, also called travel sickness, can be caused by traveling in a car, bus, boat, plane or even by swinging. It affects children as well as adults. Motion sickness results from the excessive stimulation of the labyrinthine receptors of the inner ear by certain motions. The problem is created when the motion change is rapid, irregular or continuous, such as constant speed changes in a car or plane, or the roll of a boat. Motion sickness can also be caused by confusion in the cerebellum from conflicting sensory input when visual stimulus (a moving horizon) conflicts with labyrinthine perception. Predisposing factors include tension, fear, offensive odors, or sights, sounds and feelings associated with a previous attack of motion sickness.

A weak system with weak nerves can cause motion sickness. I believe autointoxication is the main cause of motion sickness and nausea. When pregnant women have nausea and vomiting it is nature's way of cleansing the mother's body to provide a healthy environment for the baby. When children and adults experience nausea and vomiting from motion, there has to be a weakness in the system because it is not normal to have this problem.

Natural Therapy: Blood purifiers, lower bowel cleansers, fresh food and herbs to strengthen the nervous system. Nausea usually means the liver needs to be cleansed. Discourage reading, playing games, or looking down when riding in a vehicle. Good posture is essential to avoid loss of energy flow to the stomach. Create good digestion and elimination. Fresh air is very important to prevent nausea and vomiting.

Foods to Heal: Eat easily digested foods such as papaya until the stomach is strengthened and cleaned. Use proper food combining to give the stomach a chance to digest foods properly. Fruit is easily digested but must be eaten alone. Eat a lot of steamed vegetables and whole grains cooked slowly in a thermos overnight.

Vitamins and Minerals: Vitamins A and E will strengthen the mucous membranes and cells. B-complex vitamins are essential for a healthy body; they help in the assimilation, digestion and elimination of food. Vitamin B6 helps ease nausea. Vitamin C with bioflavonoids will strengthen the stomach and help in digestion. A multimineral supplement is essential. Take extra calcium, magnesium and potassium. Lack of potassium can cause incomplete digestion, constipation, nervousness and poor stomach and intestinal muscle tone.

❖

Herbal Combinations: Blood purifier, bone, digestion, glands, liver, lower bowels, nerve, potassium formulas, stress.

Single Herbs: Ginger or fennel tea will help settle the stomach. Goldenseal and gentian will clean and heal the digestive tract. Also good are lobelia extract, hops (settle a nervous stomach), kelp, papaya, peppermint tea (should always be used after vomiting), red clover, red raspberry, skullcap and wild yam.

Supplements: Acidophilus, alfalfa, mint tea, chlorophyll, green drinks, lemon and pure water, blue-green algae.

Avoid: Alcohol, cola drinks, caffeine drinks, chocolate. Avoid drinking too much soda; it leaches precious minerals and vitamins from an already weakened body. Don't drink with meals and learn to chew food well. Avoid poor food combining so the body can restore proper digestion and assimilation.

❖ MULTIPLE SCLEROSIS

Multiple sclerosis (MS) is a disease that affects the brain and spinal cord, which comprise the central nervous system. It is a degenerative state of the nervous system due to starvation of nerves and cerebrospinal cells. MS is one of the most common diseases of the nervous system in the United States. This fact is not generally known by the public because MS is not a sudden killer and it does not usually strike dramatically.

The inflammation that occurs in MS also causes hardened patches to develop at random throughout the brain and spinal cord, interfering with nerves in these areas. The damage is first noticed on the myelin coating around the nerve fibers. Myelin is the fatty material that acts as insulation around each nerve fiber. Damage to the myelin leaves the nerves exposed and the impulses from the brain center run into interference as they move along. The body attempts to repair itself and deposits hard material known as connective tissues (scars) which cannot conduct nerve impulses. The word *multiple* is used to describe the disease because of the many areas it affects and *sclerosis* is a word that means "scars."

The exact cause of multiple sclerosis is unknown, but current theories suggest that it could be a slow-acting viral infection, an autoimmune response of the nervous system, or an allergic response to an infectious agent. Other causes could include trauma, anoxia, toxins, nutritional deficiencies, vascular lesions, anorexia and stress. The following have been known to precede the onset of multiple sclerosis: emotional stress, over-work, fatigue, pregnancy and acute respiratory infections. It is also felt that endogenous, constitutional and genetic factors may also contribute.

Symptoms include weakness, loss of bladder or bowel control, slur-ring of speech, tremors and blurred or double vision. Emotional distur-bances such as mood swings, irritability, euphoria or depression also occur. Symptoms may be so mild that the patient may be unaware of them, or so bizarre that the person appears hysterical.

Diet intake seems to be the main factor in this disease. MS is com-mon in Canada, the United States and Northern Europe suggesting that a diet heavy in meat, sugar, and refined grains may be a main cause of multiple sclerosis. Animal fats, especially those found in dairy products, are linked with MS. The brain tissue of MS people have a higher satu-rated fat content than those without MS. Another theory is that infants fed cow's milk may experience nervous system disorders later in life. Breast milk has a fifth more linoleic acid than cow's milk, an acid that is essential for nervous tissues.

Natural Therapy: Blood purification and lower bowel cleansing. A change of diet is essential. A high-fiber and low-fat diet is very bene-ficial. Exercise to keep a strong circulatory system. Get plenty of sleep. Eat balanced meals. A positive attitude is essential. Correct breathing through proper exercise is important and correct sitting is vital for proper digestion, assimilation and elimination.

Foods to Heal: Fruits, vegetables, whole grains, nuts and seeds will help nourish and heal the body. Eat brown and wild rice, slowly cooked grains and steamed and raw vegetables. Use sprouts often in salads. Eat fish (cod, haddock, salmon) and fruit (apples, apricots, blackber-ries, cherries, grapes, citrus fruit, melons, peaches, pears, pineapple, plums, raspberries, strawberries), as well as all vegetables (broccoli, carrots, cabbage, cauliflower, celery).

Vitamins and Minerals: A multivitamin and mineral supplement is important. Vitamin A improves resistance to respiratory infections.

Vitamin C with bioflavonoids, B₆, B₃ and zinc are necessary for fatty acid assimilation. B-complex is very important for the nerves and especially the myelin sheath protecting the nerves. Pantothenic acid protects the myelin sheath. Folic acid, choline and inositol help in the production of lecithin. Vitamin E is vital to prevent oxidation of unsaturated fats to free radicals. Supplement with calcium and magnesium balance, potassium, phosphorus, manganese (aids in neuromuscular control), selenium, sulphur and zinc.

Herbal Combinations: Blood purifier, lower bowel cleanser, digestion, immune, nerve, stress formulas.

Single Herbs: Key herbs are garlic, ginkgo (sends circulation to the brain), hawthorn (strengthens the veins and heart), hops (strengthens the nerves), horsetail (builds bone, flesh and cartilage), Irish moss (rich in minerals), kelp, lady's slipper (brain and nerves), lobelia (cleans toxins), psyllium (food for the colon), saffron (digests fats), skullcap (feeds brain and nerves) and valerian (calms the nerves). Other vital herbs are alfalfa, black walnut (balances minerals), gentian (helps in digestion), ginger, licorice, marshmallow, myrrh, Oregon grape, slippery elm and suma.

Supplements: Essential fatty acids (evening primrose oil, salmon oil, fish oil lipids), acidophilus, lecithin (nourishes the myelin sheath around the nerves), chlorophyll and rice bran syrup (easy to digest).

Avoid: Watch for allergies and stay away from foods that cause reactions. Eliminate dairy products, meat, sugar and white flour products, caffeine, alcohol, chocolate, refined and canned foods, and white pasta products.

✤ OBESITY

When we understand how harmful being overweight can be on our bodies, and how it can predispose us to diabetes, heart disease, strokes and many other illnesses, only then will we realize how vital it is to control our eating habits. The American way of eating has given us an unhealthy appetite for damaging food. We cannot even call it food, for what we eat doesn't begin to satisfy the body's need for nutrition. If it did, our appetites would not be out of control.

When we start eating nutritional food, this alone will control our appetites because our bodies will tell us, "Hey, you have given me the vitamins and minerals I need, so I don't need anything more." The body has a natural appestat mechanism in the brain to tell us when we have eaten enough, but when it becomes distorted, we become obese. If we don't listen to our body, we essentially destroy its ability to warn us when to stop eating.

Lack of exercise also has a negative effect on the appestat mechanism. Exercise promotes circulation, an important factor in how we feel because it improves the quality of our blood. Glandular function is also improved with exercise so hormones necessary for health and appetite control are released.

Autointoxication is yet another reason for obesity. Our bodies are not able to eliminate all waste material each day so it will build up and cause us to become overweight. We need to understand the process of digestion which prepares nutrients for assimilation through the wall of the small intestines into the bloodstream. When we learn more about our bodies, we will become convinced that going on a diet is not the answer to obesity. Rather, we should change our habits when it comes to food, exercise, and how we feel about ourselves.

Natural Therapy: Blood purification and lower bowel cleansing. Lymphatic cleansing will also help clean the cells. It may take a year, but when the bloodstream and tissues are purified, the glands will function properly and you will see the weight come off naturally. Obesity is a chronic condition and it takes patience and time to overcome. Chronic diseases take a long time to acquire and take a long time to eliminate. You will feel so much better, and your whole body will be clean and healthy. A healthy body produces a healthy mind.

Foods to Heal: Fruits are cleansers of the body and vegetables are builders. Both are needed by an overweight body. Lightly steamed vegetables will provide minerals. High-fiber foods are essential. Carrot, celery, beet and apple juice are needed to feed the glands. Proper chewing will cut the appetite. Lemon juice in a glass of water first thing in the morning will clean the liver, which will help filter toxins. Green leafy vegetables, carrots, broccoli, celery, tomatoes, apples, cantaloupe, berries, melons, and plums are nutritious. Almonds, sesame seeds, seaweeds, asparagus, cabbage (red, savoy) and chives are beneficial.

❖

Use thermos-cooked whole grains for enzymes that will help in proper digestion and assimilation.

Vitamins and Minerals: These supplements are very important. The B-complex vitamins help to control appetite and the production of hydrochloric acid. B6 works with magnesium to break down proteins, fats and carbohydrates. B12 aids the body in utilizing B6, folic acid, and vitamin C. Vitamins A, C and E help the metabolism function better. Iron helps the thyroid (found in a balanced form in kelp). Herbs are rich in minerals and a multivitamin and mineral supplement is also beneficial.

Herbal Combinations: Blood purifier, cleansing, digestion, fasting formulas, glands, lower bowels, stress, nerves, weight control aid formulas.

Single Herbs: Key herbs are chickweed, glucomannan, burdock, ginkgo, ephedra, ginseng, gotu kola, fennel, hawthorn, horsetail, psyllium, saffron, skullcap, slippery elm and suma. Other important herbs are alfalfa, black cohosh, black walnut (worms and parasites may be involved), capsicum, cascara sagrada, comfrey, dandelion (cleans liver), echinacea (cleans glands), gentian (helps in digestion), licorice (helps the adrenal glands), marshmallow, papaya, parsley, passionflower, sarsaparilla (helps in hormones balance), watercress and yellow dock.

Supplements: Bee pollen, flaxseed, evening primrose oil, salmon oil, lecithin, and blue-green algae.

Avoid: All white flour and white sugar products. Eliminate chocolate, caffeine drinks, fried foods, fats and all junk food. Avoid salty food as it puts a strain on the thyroid gland.

❖ OSTEOPOROSIS

Osteoporosis is a metabolic bone disorder which slows down the rate of bone formation and accelerates the rate of bone resorption, causing loss of bone mass. The bones affected by this disease lose essential calcium and phosphate salts and become porous like a honeycomb. As a result they are brittle and vulnerable to fractures, even without serious falls or injuries. In fact, the presence of osteoporosis is usually discovered by the occurrence of spontaneous fractures of the hip, spine or long bones. It cannot be detected even with x-rays until 50 percent of the bone has been lost.

Osteoporosis is most common in women due to long-term calcium losses during pregnancies and menstruation. They also have thinner bones than men. The disease does occur in men, but because men have heavier bones they are more resistant to osteoporosis, at least until their later years.

Studies done by Dr. Kervran, a European scientist, found that fractures do not knit when there are high amounts of calcium present in bones but little or no silica. However, he noted that bones knit extremely well when there is an abundance of silica present but little calcium. Kervran found that silica is the first most important supplement in bone health, manganese the second and potassium the third. Kervran feels that a significant percentage of bone breaks and fractures could be avoided altogether if sufficient silica is present. Horsetail and oatstraw have high amounts of silica, manganese, copper and other nutrients.

Natural Therapy: Blood purification and lower bowel cleansing will help improve digestion. A change of diet is required and short fasts will improve assimilation of nutrients. Exercise will help control bone loss. Regular exercise improves calcium absorption and stimulates bone formation. The best exercise is walking briskly, or an aerobic type exercise where you can get your heart beat up. A minitrampoline is excellent when you use your upper body to reach your ideal heart rate.

Foods to Heal: Whole grains, buckwheat and brown rice are high in magnesium and silica. Green leafy vegetables, salads and lightly steamed vegetables are nutritious. Millet is easy to digest. Almonds, soybeans, sesame seeds, lima beans, red and white beans are high in magnesium. Sprouts will help in digestion and the assimilation of essential minerals. Foods high in calcium and low in phosphorus are almonds, sesame seeds, kale, leafy greens, kelp, Irish moss and parsley.

Vitamins and Minerals: Vitamins C and D increase the absorption of calcium and other vital minerals. Fluorine, found naturally in herbs, prevents bone loss. Phosphorus is vital to calcium and the ratio between the two is important. We get too much phosphorus in meat, cola drinks and processed foods. Magnesium helps prevent calcification by keeping calcium in solution so it can be absorbed. Half the amount of magnesium to that of calcium is needed to aid in proper calcium absorption. Silica is essential along with all minerals.

Herbal Combinations: Bone (rich in silica), digestion, glands.

Single Herbs: Key herbs are alfalfa, black walnut (help balance minerals), comfrey, horsetail, Irish moss, kelp, oatstraw, red clover and slippery elm. Other important herbs are dandelion, echinacea, garlic, ginger, ginseng, goldenseal (heals the digestive tract), hawthorn, licorice, lobelia, marshmallow, papaya, plantain and sarsaparilla.

Supplements: Evening primrose oil, salmon oil, acidophilus, chlorophyll, lecithin.

Avoid: All sugar products, caffeine drinks, soft drinks, alcohol, all refined grains.

✦ PARKINSON'S DISEASE

Parkinson's is a degenerative disease of the nervous system which is characterized by tremors and stiffness of muscles. Although the cause of Parkinson's disease is not known, there is an imbalance of two chemicals, dopamine and acetylcholine, seen in patients. Dopamine carries messages from one nerve cell to another and when the body cannot produce it, the symptoms of Parkinson's appear. Because the brain and nervous system are very sensitive to toxins and a lack of nutrients, many health practitioners believe that malnutrition is the cause of this disease. Other causes may be the many medications that are given to older people, a viral infection, or carbon monoxide poisoning.

Over sixty thousand older adults develop drug-induced Parkinson's each year. Drugs are prescribed in excessive amounts to the elderly, especially for chronic anxiety and gastrointestinal complaints. Stelazine, a powerful antipsychotic tranquilizer that is prescribed to calm the intestinal tract, can induce Parkinson's. The irony is that yet another drug is given to control the disease, when a prescription drug is what caused it in the first place.

Levodopa is a drug that is given to treat Parkinson's. When levodopa is taken alone, avoid foods and vitamins that contain vitamin B6. This vitamin can destroy the effectiveness of the drug. B6 is one of the vitamins that protects the system from nerve disorders. The following drugs can block the action of dopamine and cause the symptoms of Parkinson's disease: Phenothiazines, droperidol, haloperidol, reserpine (found in heart drugs such as diupres, enduronyl, and hydropres), chlorprothixene, thiothixene, methyldopa, metoclopramide and lithium. It pays to know what drugs you are taking and what their side effects can induce.

Natural Therapy: The first natural therapy is to look for the cause, whether it is medications, heavy metal poisoning, diet or nutritional deficiencies. A hair analysis is important to determine metal poisoning. Blood purification is also therapeutic. Improve digestion so the nutrients can circulate to the brain. Use a natural chelation program to dissolve toxins on the artery walls. Exercise is important and a positive attitude is vital for improvement.

Foods to Heal: Brewer's yeast, wheat germ, wheat bran, molasses, honey, and whole grains (cooked in thermos for digestion and retention of the B-complex vitamins). Whole wheat, buckwheat and millet are easily digested. Use yellow corn meal, barley, brown rice. Fresh fruit and vegetables are necessary. Use safflower oil and lemon juice as a dressing on green salads every day. Almonds and sesame seeds are high in calcium and magnesium. Sprouts will provide nutrients that are easily digested. Eat all natural foods.

Vitamins and Minerals: Multivitamin and mineral supplements are essential. Make sure they are being assimilated. Vitamins A, C, and E are vital for the immune system along with selenium and zinc. The B-complex vitamins feed the nerves and brain. Take extra B_6, B_{12}, and niacin. Calcium, magnesium and silica are essential. Herbal bone combinations will provide these, as well as other essential minerals such as manganese.

Herbal Combinations: Blood purifier, bone, chelation, digestion, liver and gallbladder, lower bowels, nerve and stress formulas.

Single Herbs: Key herbs are ginkgo (strengthens the brain and nervous system) gotu kola (rebuilds energy food for the brain), hawthorn (for veins and heart), hops (nerve food), horsetail, kelp (feeds and cleans veins), lady's slipper (helps tremors), lobelia (cleanser and relaxer), passionflower (helps the nerves), red clover (cleans the blood of toxins), skullcap (settles the brain), suma (strengthens the whole body), valerian (relaxer) and wood betony (good for pain). Other vital herbs are alfalfa, black cohosh, black walnut, burdock, capsicum, chaparral, comfrey, echinacea, garlic, gentian (cleans the entire digestive system), ginger, ginseng, goldenseal, mistletoe, St. John's wort and yellow dock.

Supplements: Chlorophyll, lecithin, blue-green algae, aloe vera, green drinks, wheat grass juice, evening primrose oil, salmon oil (may help to reduce tremors).

Avoid: Avoid cooking in aluminum pots and eliminate antacids, baking powder, pickles, relishes and some cheeses. Aluminum can also be present in soft drinks and beers in uncoated aluminum cans. It is also found in antidepressants. Avoid all drugs and stimulants; they destroy the nervous system and the brain. Caffeine, tobacco, tea, cola drinks, chocolate, a high-meat diet, alcohol, sugar and white flour products. They contain no nutrients and leach nutrients that are essential for the brain and nervous system such as calcium, and B-complex vitamins.

❖ PARASITES AND WORMS

Parasites and worms are becoming a real problem in the United States. Even if your surroundings are highly sanitized, the inside of our bodies still need to be clean. The diet of the American people encourages parasites and worms. A diet rich in fat, starch and sugar provides food that these scavengers live on. A well-nourished body, on the other hand, will provide an environment in which parasites are unable to thrive.

One current problem that is sweeping across the country is a parasite that causes intestinal infections. It is called *Giardia lamblia* and has now become the number one cause of waterborne disease in the United States. Tapeworm infection is also increasing by leaps and bounds. It has been linked with Americans' increasing fondness for raw and rare beef. Baiantidium parasite comes from pigs and causes intestinal infections in humans, a compelling reason why pork should be left out of the diet. The painful and serious disease called amoebic dysentery results from amoeba that destroy the intestinal lining of the humans. This can cause the body to become dehydrated and eventually cause bleeding and ulceration in the bowel.

Flatworms and roundworms are other parasites that cause serious damage and can often kill their hosts. There is one type of flatworm called a fluke which lives and grows quite large in the intestines, liver, lungs or blood of animals and man. Another common worm, the tapeworm, absorbs digested foods from its host. The hookworm is the most harmful type. It lives in the intestines and feeds on the blood of the host.

Trichinosis is a disease that comes from eating pork. The trichina is a tiny worm that infects pigs. The larvae, after burrowing into the intestinal wall of the pig, then enters its blood vessels. The blood carries the larvae to the muscles fiber and lives. Then when humans eat the pork, the cycle begins again in the human body. Symptoms of trichinosis are headaches, fever, sore muscles, swollen eyes, and even painful breathing. These symptoms are similar to other diseases so people do not even realize that they could have internal worms.

It has been theorized that cancer may also be caused by a parasite. In her book *The Conquest of Cancer*, Dr. Virginia Livingston-Wheeler, M. D. explains that a parasite called the progenitor cryptocids begins as the lepra or tuberular bacilli and changes form to become the cancer parasite. She says that this microbe is present in all of our cells, and it is only our immune systems that keep it suppressed. When our immune system is weakened, either by poor diet, infected food, or old age, this microbe gains a foothold and starts cancer cells growing into tumors.

Natural Therapy: The most therapeutic thing that can be done is blood purification with a lower bowel cleansing. The body needs to be cleaned and purified. The body is a wonderful machine and when nourished and treated properly will not harbor these scavengers. When there are sufficient amounts of healthy bile, the parasites and worms, along with their larvae and eggs, are neutralized and evacuated rapidly out of the body. For this reason the digestive system also needs to be cleaned and healed. Parasites and worms cannot live in a clean body and they especially do not like minerals. Herbs have high amounts of minerals and other elements that will help eliminate them. Sometimes people become discouraged when they try to live

❖

on a more wholesome diet or try to go on a cleansing purge. It is hard for them to stay on it because the parasites within are crying for the kind of junk foods upon which they live and grow. It is probably wise to clean the body of the parasites first. Since parasites cling to the mucus in which they live, the body cannot be made well even in a fasting or semi-fasting situation.

Foods to Heal: Garlic and onion are two of the best foods to eradicate worms and parasites because of their high sulfur content. Grind and use pumpkin seeds often on cereals—they kill worms and parasites and are especially beneficial for children. Grated raw beets will also kill worms. Carrots, scrubbed, washed and eaten with the skin left on, are rich in organic minerals and act as worm killers. Figs and fig juice, especially white juice, paralyze any worms. Papaya seeds are effective for expelling worms. Pomegranates also kill worms.

Vitamins and Minerals: Vitamins A, B, C, D and E all build-up the immune system and encourage a healthy digestive system. A multi-mineral supplement containing selenium, silica and zinc discourages parasites and worms.

Herbal Combinations: Blood purifier, digestion, immune, liver, lower bowels, parasites and worms, potassium.

Single Herbs: Key herbs are aloe vera, black walnut and burdock (equal parts for purging out parasites and worms), chaparral (eliminates worms), echinacea (cleans the lymphatics), garlic (kills worms), goldenseal (kills worms and parasites), horsetail (rich in minerals so discourages worms), kelp (high in minerals, cleansing), papaya (kills worms), parsley (cleans kidneys), psyllium (cleans colon), red clover (blood cleanser), senna (keeps colon clean), wormwood (kills worms) and yellow dock (rich in iron to kill parasites and their eggs). Other beneficial herbs are alfalfa, buchu, catnip, cornsilk, hops, gotu kola, lady's slipper, lobelia, pau d'arco, peppermint, queen of the meadow, St. John's wort, wood betony and yarrow.

Supplements: Acidophilus, chlorophyll (cleans blood), bentonite, chelated cell salts, glucomannan, spirulina, diatomaceous earth, hydrochloric acid supplements and pancreatic enzymes.

Avoid: A high-meat diet, a high-fat diet, and sugar products of all kinds. Also avoid constipation. It encourages worms and parasites.

✣ Periodontal Disease

According to the U.S. Public Health Service, 98 percent of all Americans fall prey to dental disease. The American Dental Association relates that by retirement, the average senior citizen has only five teeth left and 40 percent are wearing dentures. In an advanced modern society, with the latest in technology and sophisticated knowledge, why do we have such poor dental health?

The definition of periodontal is "of the tissues surrounding and supporting the teeth." One of the first signs of periodontal disease is bleeding gums. When gums are inflamed, this condition is known as gingivitis. Poor diet is the major culprit in gingivitis. Lack of vitamin C can cause scurvy-like symptoms, which include bleeding gums and loose teeth.

Good oral hygiene is also necessary. Flossing daily and brushing from the base of the teeth toward the crown can do much to clean away plaque. Plaque, a film on the teeth where bacteria flourish, can harden into a rock-like substance known as tartar. Tartar accumulates at the base of the tooth where the gum line meets. If the plaque isn't brushed off daily, the tartar irritates the gums further and causes more bleeding. The bacteria loosen the teeth from the gums and migrate lower, where they form pus pockets. This extremely dangerous condition is known as pyorrhea. Pus discharges into the mouth and the teeth will actually loosen from the sockets. The roots are destroyed and the teeth are extracted, hence the need for dentures. This entire collection of symptoms is known as periodontal disease.

Dental experts feel that loss of bone mass beneath the teeth is the major contributor to dental problems. It is called osteoporosis of the jaws. A strong bone mass is important beneath the teeth. If not, it will be easier for bacteria to get in and cause further damage.

Natural Therapy: Blood purification (toxins in the blood stream can settle in the gum area). For the assimilation of nutrients vital for strong teeth and gums sufficient hydrochloric acid is necessary. If stomach acids are low, it can contribute to poor teeth.

Foods to Heal: Foods high in bone- and teeth-strengthening fluorine are leaf lettuce, cabbage, radishes, egg whites, beets, lentils, parsnips and

❖

whole grains. Foods high in silicon to assist calcium assimilation are Boston and bibb lettuce, parsnip, asparagus, rice bran, onions, spinach, cucumber, strawberry, leeks, savoy cabbage, sunflower seeds, Swiss chard, pumpkin, celery, cauliflower, cherry, apricot, fresh, millet, grapes, apples and sweet potatoes. Foods high in calcium are sesame seeds, collard and kale leaves, almonds, soybeans, mustard, spinach, filbert, chickpeas, white beans, pinto beans, dried figs, sunflower seeds, whole grains.

Vitamins and Minerals: Vitamin A nourishes mucous membranes. B-complex vitamins are necessary for bones and teeth. Vitamin C with bioflavonoids prevents infections. Vitamin D works with calcium for strong bones. Vitamin E protects by enhancing oxygen to cells. All minerals are vital for bone and teeth health. Scientific research has shown what a crucial function silicon has in calcium metabolism, bone formation, normal growth and prevention of osteoporosis and jaw bone loss. (Herbal calcium contains all minerals for bone health.) The calcium in milk cannot be assimilated properly because of the nutrients lost in pasteurizing and homogenizing. Selenium and zinc are important in healing bones.

Herbal Combinations: Bone, immune, nerve, potassium, stress.

Single Herbs: Black walnut (strengthens teeth—you can brush with it), comfrey (heals and repairs gums), goldenseal (add black walnut and brush teeth), horsetail (contains silica and other minerals to grow bone mass), kelp (minerals for healthy gums and teeth), oak bark (heals and strengthens gums, brush teeth with it), oatstraw, pau d'arco, slippery elm and yellow dock.

Supplements: Chlorophyll, evening primrose oil, salmon oil, tea tree oil (put some on toothpaste), coenzyme Q_{10}, germanium, hydrochloric acid and pancreatic enzyme supplements.

Avoid: Toothbrushes accumulate germs so you can rinse with alcohol to kill bacteria. Use dental floss! Avoid all sugar products as they invite bacteria. Tobacco causes bone loss. Soft drinks contain phosphorus and so contribute to an imbalance in the calcium/phosphorus ratio. Avoid all products that will harm the immune system.

✤ PREGNANCY

Pregnancy can be a very happy experience if the mother's body is free from toxins. Toxins can cause nausea and hormonal imbalances. Toxemia is common and a very dangerous condition for both the mother and baby. Hormonal imbalances are due to constipation, with the liver failing to eliminate toxins faster than they accumulate. Even before becoming pregnant, parents should learn more about their bodies and the importance of a healthy diet as well as the dangers of drugs, caffeine and alcohol. Even over-the-counter drugs like aspirin seem harmless but can cause birth defects in the early months of pregnancy.

There are many complaints of pregnancy which can be remedied naturally without resorting to drugs or over-the-counter remedies. Constipation, morning sickness, leg cramps, indigestion, fatigue, swollen ankles and varicose veins or backache are a few of the problems that pregnant women encounter. Pregnancy increases the body's need for nutrients. Eating a healthy diet will provide nutrients for a healthy and happy baby. Women on who consume large amounts of junk food have a higher incidence of difficult labors, premature babies, birth defects, infections, hemorrhages, nursing problems and problems during their pregnancy.

Natural Therapy: It is essential to adopt a natural diet to provide nutrients for mother and baby alike. A healthy body doesn't just happen—you have to work at it. Learn the importance of food in obtaining vitamins, minerals and nutrients that assist the development of a healthy fetus. Blood purification is essential; using herbs and green drinks will help nourish the mother and baby. Exercise will help supply oxygen for the fetus as well as strengthen the mother for easier birth. Sitz baths are common in Europe for pregnant women. In fact, most bathrooms have a special sink for sitz baths. The warm and cold water brings increased circulation the pelvic area and it is felt that sitz baths help almost every problem of a pregnant woman.

Foods to Heal: Protein is essential, and grains, buckwheat and millet are complete proteins. A high-fiber diet will keep the bowels functioning properly. A supply of vitamins and minerals is needed for mother and baby. Grains, nuts and seeds contain properties that help increase immunity to disease. Oats, yellow corn meal, barley, and all grains are good. Seeds are high in calcium and other minerals; flax, sesame, chia and pumpkin are the best. Vegetables are important, fresh and steamed. Potatoes, yams, squash, green beans can be steamed. Eat raw salads every day. Fruits are cleansers of the body.

Vitamins and Minerals: Take a multivitamin and mineral for ideal nutrition. Vitamin A promotes growth and protects against toxins. B-complex protects the body from exhaustion and irritability. Extra B_6 controls swelling and nausea. Vitamin B_{12} creates more energy. The B vitamins strengthen the brain and heart. Vitamin C complex helps to enhance contractions and minimize stretch marks. It protects against viruses. It will protect the growing embryo from virus particles in the mother's tissues. Vitamin D is essential to help calcium absorb. It is vital for bone and teeth development and helps jaw bones develop so the teeth have room for proper growth. Vitamin E reduces the body's need for oxygen, strengthens the circulatory system and helps to prevent miscarriage.

Minerals are essential; even if one mineral is lacking it could cause birth defects. Calcium is required more during pregnancy but a deficiency is caused by a high-meat diet. Calcium is needed with vitamin D for proper bone development. Iron builds the blood and is essential for the baby's liver. Yellow dock contains 40 percent easily assimilated iron. Silicon helps the body utilize calcium. Magnesium works with calcium. Selenium, potassium and zinc protect the immune system.

Herbal Combinations: Blood purifiers, calcium or bone formulas, immune formulas, digestion, lower bowel (small doses to keep the bowels open), nerve formulas (contain nutrients for nervous system), stress and special formulas to use the last six weeks of pregnancy for a safer and easier delivery. Some of the herbs contained in them are black cohosh, red raspberry, squaw vine, blessed thistle, pennyroyal and lobelia.

Single Herbs: Alfalfa contains protein, vitamins, minerals, and is also a blood cleanser. It is high in vitamin K which clots the blood and prevents hemorrhage. Red raspberry tea is high in iron and calcium. Mint teas will help with nausea. Dandelion and kelp are high in essential vitamins and minerals. Dandelion cleans and protects the liver while kelp cleans the veins and provides nourishment. Also important are cascara sagrada (small amounts), ginger (helps settle stomach), oatstraw, papaya, marshmallow and yellow dock. Other beneficial herbs are garlic, hawthorn, hops, skullcap and slippery elm (rich in protein and nourishing).

Supplements: Acidophilus, chlorophyll, evening primrose oil, salmon oil, green drinks, wheat grass juice, blue-green algae.

Avoid: Alcohol passes freely through the placenta and is very toxic to the fetus. Stay away from chemicals such as preservatives, additives, food colorings, pesticides, and any unnatural substance like MSG. Chemicals overwork the liver. Drugs should also be avoided. Aspirin interferes with the clotting of blood. Antibiotics interfere with the production of RNA and protein, and could cause damage to the fetus. Other problems with drugs are jaundice, respiratory problems, deformed limbs, mental retardation and digestive problems. If you smoke, stop. Carbon monoxide prevents the intake of oxygen in the fetus and could cause birth defects, stunted growth, low birth weight and hyperactive children. It usually does cause premature births. Avoid sugar, white flour products and fried foods because they rob the body of nutrients.

❖ PREMENSTURAL SYNDROME

Premenstrual syndrome (PMS) is not a disease nor a mental disorder, but is often treated as such. Over 150 symptoms have been linked to this disorder, the most common being depression, irritability, faintness, restlessness, sluggishness, impatience, lethargy, delusion, indecisiveness, dizziness, nervousness, anxiety, swelling of breasts, feet swelling, constipation, hemorrhoids, skin eruptions, migraines, backaches and puffiness. The imbalance in the system could stem from genetic predisposition, an organic malfunction, a vitamin or mineral deficiency, stress, drugs or chemicals, or a combination of these. Many of these symptoms can be linked to nutritional deficiencies.

The liver is responsible for regulating hormonal balances. The liver is responsible for filtering blood levels of estradiol, the unfavorable type of estrogen, but someties it can build up in the body. When this excess estrogen is allowed to enter the bloodstream, it travels to the brain and nervous system and causes depression and bizarre mental manifestations. Constipation is the main cause of liver being unable to filter out the excess, unwanted estrogen.

Food cravings, unusual outbreaks of temper, and bizarre thinking affect many women within the PMS interval. Desire for sweets or high-carbohydrate foods, caffeine drinks, chocolate, and all kinds of junk food are manifested at this time.

Some women who are accustomed to drinking alcoholic beverages often go on "binges" just before their periods. Low estrogen levels, naturally occurring during the PMS period, heighten the effect of alcohol. The drinker suffers a stronger reaction from the same amount ingested. This alleviates depression. The physical complications, related to alcohol use, are too dangerous to ignore. Alcohol is often used as a tranquilizer to relieve PMS discomfort. If relief is found, the results are temporary and usually lead to further problems.

Natural Therapy: Blood purification, lower bowel formulas, and a cleansing fast will help the liver eliminate toxins that cause PMS symptoms. The body will heal itself when given the natural nutrients. Women with severe autointoxication have serious problems. It will take patience and endurance to implement and follow a nutritional diet to clean and build the body back to health. Nervine therapy using herbs to strengthen the nervous system is one of the best methods to help with PMS. Physical exercise is also very helpful before and during menstruation. Vigorous exercise stimulates circulation and deep breathing and improves the supply of nutrients throughout the system. Stress intensifies symptoms of PMS so it needs to be dealt with. In many canses, the mind can determine the health of the body.

Foods to Heal: Food high in fiber and fruits, vegetables, grains, nuts and seeds are healing. Brown rice and wild rice are excellent. Try cooking millet and brown rice together. Oats, whole wheat, yellow corn meal, buckwheat and millet are all high in fiber, vitamins and minerals (use thermos cooking to retain nutrients and enzymes). Yellow vegetables help keep the bowels clean. Salads, using leaf lettuce, cabbage, carrots, broccoli, and all raw vegetables are very nourishing. Also use sprouts in salads and in sandwiches. Nuts are high in protein, calcium and fiber. Almonds are the best, and pecans, cashews, walnuts, and filberts are also good. Grind and use seed such as chia, flax, sunflower and sesame which are very high in calcium. Foods rich in magnesium are beans, grains and dark green vegetables.

Vitamins and Minerals: Vitamin A helps to regulate the female cycle and protect the glands. B-complex vitamins combat fatigue and help to reduce sugar cravings, weight fluctuation and bloating. B-complex vitamins are vital to provide the liver the necessary material to detoxify excess estrogen in the body and prevent hormonal imbalance. B_6 helps in treating tension, aggression, depression and irritability. It also acts as a natural diuretic. B_2 is needed during stress; lack of it can cause depression, hysteria, trembling and fatigue. B vitamins are needed daily. Vitamin C with bioflavonoids helps strengthen the walls of the small blood vessels and the immune system. It relieves stress and acts as a natural diuretic when menstrual flow is too heavy. Vitamin E helps ease the symptoms of PMS, relieves pain, helps with cramps, inhibits breast tenderness and increases resistance to stress. It is important in the production and proper metabolism of the sex hormones.

Minerals are vital. Calcium and magnesium deficiencies can cause headaches, nervous disorders, fluid retention and pain. About ten days before menstruation, calcium levels drop and remain low until the period is over. Calcium and magnesium relieve cramps, calm and act as blood clotting agents. They work with vitamin D for absorption. Iodine is necessary for thyroxin to break down estrogen. Kelp is an herb high in natural iodine and other essential minerals. Selenium and zinc prevent toxins from accumulating. Potassium and silicon help regulate the body's needs and helps in assimilation of calcium.

Herbal Combinations: Anemia, bone, digestion, female formulas, glandular, nerve and PMS formulas. Lower bowel and liver formulas will help clean the body.

Single Herbs: Key herbs are black cohosh, blessed thistle, damiana, dong quai (helps in all menstrual problems), false unicorn, hops, kelp, lobelia, red clover (cleans blood and liver), red raspberry (the greatest

herb for all women's problems), sarsaparilla (helps balance hormones), skullcap (calms the nerves and brain), squaw vine, saw palmetto (balances hormones), valerian, wood betony and yellow dock
(rich in iron). Other important herbs are alfalfa, burdock, chamomile
(eases pain in cramps), gentian (helps digestive system), gotu kola
(feeds the brain), hawthorn (circulation), licorice (hormone balancer)
and parsley (helps in water retention).

Supplements: Evening primrose oil, salmon oil, spirulina, chlorophyll,
acidophilus, blue-green algae.

Avoid: Foods high in refined sugars and fats as well as highly processed
foods full of chemicals. Salt causes irritability, breast tenderness and
water retention. A combination of sugar and salt maximizes problems
with pain and swelling. Avoid diuretics, they cause loss of potassium
and magnesium. Caffeine leaches calcium so stay away from coffee,
black tea, chocolate and soda pop. They also contribute to breast lumps
and swelling. Nicotine destroys nutrients and produces symptoms the
same as caffeine does. Alcohol destroys the liver and bloodstream.

For any problems with the reproductive system, it would be wise
to avoid all food that relate to the reproductive system of animals, or
food that contains artificial hormones. This includes milk and all
milk products, all meat of animals that have been raised on hormones. Chlorinated water destroys the benefits of vitamin E and
causes hormone imbalance. Avoid birth control pills; they deplete the
body of B-vitamins, especially folic acid, B$_6$, and B$_{12}$.

✤ Prostate Problems

The prostate is a male gland about the size of a walnut that lies
between the rectum and urethra. The function of the prostate is the production of the sperm cells. Life itself is a part of this gland. It is also
thought that specific hormones and enzymes are manufactured there.
The prostate provides a passageway for urine and when inflammation
strikes, it can cause pain and discomfort.

Men usually eat a lot of animal products, and this can lead to a long-
term putrefaction, an autointoxication that gradually builds up in the
body. The prostate is especially vulnerable to bacterial infections that
seep in from toxic waste emanating from the colon.

Prostatitis is inflammation of the prostate which can affect young as well as adult men. Prostate hypertrophy is labeled a condition of aging. It is a swelling and enlargement of the prostate usually seen in males over the age of forty. Research on prostate problems with males who suffer from this disease show their diets are usually low in fatty acids (nuts, seeds, salmon oil) and vitamin C, bioflavonoids, vitamin E and zinc.

Prostate cancer is a devastating disease that medical doctors treat with surgery and hormone therapy. This disease is also linked to deficient diets. Prostate cancer, along with other diseases, first appeared in the twentieth century. Overly processed food has depleted vitamins and minerals from the diet. Zinc is one example. The prostate needs zinc, selenium and lecithin. A high-fat diet clogs up the liver and gall bladder and causes constipation, which eventually creates autointoxication.

Natural Therapy: Blood purification, lower bowel cleansing, and sitz bath. Sit in a tub of hot water with a horsetail infusion (put in a cloth packet to avoid a mess). This can be done twenty to thirty minutes twice a day. A change of diet is needed, with less meat and more vegetables, fruit, nuts, seeds.

Foods to Heal: Pumpkin seeds contain fatty acids and are beneficial for intestinal worms. Sesame, chia and flaxseeds are also high in fatty acids. Eat nuts, such as almonds, pine, cashew, pistachio and pecans. Whole grains (cooked in thermos) are rich in minerals and B vitamins. Green salads containing sprouts, parsley and watercress are beneficial. Steamed vegetables such as winter squash, carrots, asparagus, broccoli and cabbage are high in minerals. Dried beans, endives, hazelnuts, dried peas, brown rice, soy flour, cashews, Brazil nuts, corn, and sunflower seeds are all high in magnesium which helps prevent infections. Water is very important; drink about eight glasses a day. This dilutes urine to help avoid bacterial growth in the bladder and helps flush the prostate urethra.

Vitamins and Minerals: Vitamins A and E protect against infections. Nutritionists have found vitamin C very effective in correcting prostate infections, but large amounts are needed. A multimineral supplement is vital to help to avoid infections, especially magnesium, potassium, silicon and zinc.

Herbal Combinations: Blood purifier, chelation, glands, immune formulas, infection, kidney, lower bowels, pain, prostate formulas.

Single Herbs: Key herbs are alfalfa, buchu, comfrey, cornsilk, damiana, garlic, ginseng, goldenseal, horsetail, juniper berries, kelp, parsley, red clover, saw palmetto (helps to shrink prostate to relieve pain) and uva ursi. Other beneficial herbs are black cohosh, black walnut, blessed thistle, burdock, chaparral, capsicum, dandelion, echinacea, false unicorn, ginger, hawthorn, hops, lady's slipper, marshmallow pau d'arco (blood purifier), red clover, St. John's wort, wood betony, yarrow and yellow dock.

Supplements: Bee pollen (good for prostatitis), essential fatty acids (safflower, sunflower, olive oils), evening primrose oil, salmon oil, chlorophyll and lecithin (assists in functions of EFAs and also dissolves fats to prevent cholesterol). Royal jelly is good. Germanium and coenzyme Q_{10} are beneficial for circulation.

Avoid: Alcohol, caffeine and nicotine have a negative effect on the prostate. Coffee is bad, even if it is decaffeinated. The aromatic oils in coffee weakens the prostate. Once the prostate becomes enlarged or even slightly irritated it becomes susceptible to the effects of alcohol, strong coffee, tea, uric acid in meat, and drugs. Avoid a high-fat diet, especially fried foods (they create free radicals which destroy cells).

✤ RAYNAUD'S DISEASE

Raynaud's disease involves poor circulation to the hands and feet. Basically, it is a disease of the small arteries so there is interference with the blood circulation to the fingers and toes. They become very sensitive to cold. After exposure to stress or cold, the skin of the fingers changes colors from blanched to blue or red. Numbness and tingling may also occur. These symptoms can be relieved by warmth.

This disease was first discovered and explained by a Frenchman 100 years ago when he described a tightening of the arteries extending to the hands and feet. When they become cold there is less blood sent to the skin, and so the outlying arteries contract accordingly. Some drugs that affect the blood vessels such as antihypertensives and channel blockers can also cause this disease.

Natural Therapy: Blood purification, and circulatory therapy. Keep the hands and feet warm at all times and avoid injury to them. Change your diet, adding raw vegetables and eating less fatty, fried foods, and meat. Add as much natural food to the diet as possible.

Foods to Heal: A high-fiber diet, using whole grains, freshly ground to retain all the nutrients. All the ingredients in grains work together to prevent diseases. Millet, buckwheat, barley, whole wheat and rye are all good grains. Beans, and lentils are very good. Use sprouts in salads and eat fresh and steamed vegetables, lots of fresh fruit, nuts and seeds.

Vitamins and Minerals: Vitamin E is very important to improve circulation. Vitamin B-complex is important for liver health in the metabolism of fat. Niacin improves circulation by dilating the small arteries. Vitamin C with bioflavonoids will help strengthen and clean the small arteries.

Herbal Combinations: Blood purifiers, chelation, digestion, heart, potassium, stress formulas.

Single Herbs: Key herbs are butcher's broom (improves circulation and strengthens the veins), capsicum (cleans veins), garlic, ginkgo (improves circulation), hawthorn (strengthens the arteries and heart), ephedra, ginger, ginseng, gotu kola, horsetail, parsley, saffron and skullcap. Other important herbs are black cohosh, bugleweed, blessed thistle, burdock, cramp bark, dandelion, lobelia, mistletoe, oatstraw, passionflower, rose hips and yarrow.

Supplements: Chlorophyll (strengthens veins and arteries), lecithin (prevents fatty deposits), essential fatty acids, evening primrose oil, salmon oil, safflower and sunflower oils, glucomannan, germanium and coenzyme Q_{10}.

Avoid: Injury to hands and feet. If the disease is severe maybe a warm climate would be best. Avoid all food and beverages that interfere with health and good circulation: alcohol, coffee, tea, cola drinks. Avoid sugar; it robs vital nutrients necessary for good circulation. Avoid certain drugs that interfere with the body's natural healing process.

❖ RHEUMATIC FEVER

Millions of people are treated annually for strep infections to prevent rheumatic fever, a disease that rarely exists in modern times Penicillin,

❖

the treatment for this disease, is more of a health hazard than the disease. Those who risk this disease are people living in poverty and unsanitary conditions. Studies have shown that rheumatic fever is related to the density of children per room. Fresh air, good nutrition and clean sanitation are lacking and seem to go hand in hand with this disease.

Rheumatic fever is caused from a streptococcal bacteria, causing infection with strep throat, tonsillitis, scarlet fever or ear infection. If left untreated, it can affect the heart, brain and joints. It can be a serious disease, but in most cases these symptoms can be treated naturally with antibiotic herbs. It is very seldom that children get this disease. The symptoms are pain, inflammation, stiffness, joint pain and fever. Skin rash has also been seen. After the body has been weakened with rheumatic fever, it can occur again. If rheumatic fever does occur, in my opinion it is better to use antibiotics to clear up the infection, and then clean and purify the body of the drugs and toxins after it is over. This way you can avoid permanent kidney or heart damage.

Natural Therapy: Blood purification, lower bowel cleansing, juice fasting, enemas, garlic/catnip. While the acute symptoms last, use only fresh citrus juices and herbal teas (red raspberry, peppermint, catnip) to assist the body in healing. Use herbal extracts that will assimilate into the bloodstream for a speedy recovery.

Foods to Heal: Ground seeds such as sesame, sunflower, and pumpkin will help keep the body clean and prevent serious infections. Brown rice and millet (thermos cooked) are nutritious. Vegetables such as carrots, sweet potatoes, parsley, sprouts, turnips, broccoli, brussels sprouts, cauliflower, winter squash, cabbage and onions should be a regular part of the diet. Fruit is cleansing so eat apricots, citrus fruits, apples, berries, and grapes.

Vitamins and Minerals: Vitamin A is a protection to the mucous membranes and prevents harm from germs and viruses. Vitamin B-complex is needed for healing and building the immune system. Vitamin C with bioflavonoids helps eliminate infection, reduce pain, and flush toxins from the body. Vitamin C works with A for healing and absorption of calcium and minerals. Vitamin E provides oxygen for cell cleansing and health. Multiminerals are important for all minerals are needed for healing. Do a liquid for fast assimilation and take extra calcium, magnesium, potassium selenium, silicon and zinc.

Herbal Combinations: Blood purifiers, bone formulas, colds and flu, immune, pain and stress formulas.

Single Herbs: Key herbs are alfalfa and mint teas (hot), catnip, chamomile (soothing and calming), cascara sagrada (opens the bowels), echinacea (cleans the lymphatics), garlic (natural antibiotic), ginger (baths are good), goldenseal (relieves itching and a natural antibiotic), hops (relaxing for the nerves), pau d'arco (cleans and protects the liver), peppermint (settles the stomach and helps the body eliminate toxins), pleurisy root (helps in the pain), red raspberry and skullcap. Other important herbs are capsicum, eyebright, lady's slipper, lobelia, mullein, red clover, rose hips, saffron, yarrow and yellow dock.

Supplements: Chlorophyll, essential fatty acids, evening primrose oil, salmon oil, safflower, sunflower seed, olive oil (cold pressed) and instant vitamin and minerals.

Avoid: This acute disease is a cleansing and healing of the body during which the stomach accumulates toxins squeezed out of the cells. If normal eating continues this stops the natural cleansing and healing process. This will cause rheumatic fever to recur or cause damage to organs of the body. Avoid all sugar products as they deplete vital nutrients from the body. Stay away from all white flour products, white rice, refined grains, potato chips, fried foods, bacon, sausage, ham, smoked meat and fish, hot dogs, salami, bologna, cold cuts, corned beef, chocolate, caffeine drinks and cola drinks. Avoid all food with preservatives and additives.

✤ SENILITY

Senility seems to go along with aging. Drugs are one of the main causes of senility, along with a lack of nutrients. Older people are given drugs in larger amounts than their body can excrete. They are given tranquilizers, high blood pressure drugs, and all kinds of drugs for nervous system disorders. These affect the brain and nervous system. It is felt by many health doctors that prescription drugs should be given less frequently and in smaller amounts. They feel the elderly are being drugged into senility.

❖

The brain is the most sensitive organ and reacts to poor nutrition, drugs, air pollution, and bad water. When a brain neuron dies it can never be replaced. It can be destroyed by drugs, alcohol and drugs together, concussion, stroke or inflammation. A lack of nutrients to the brain can also cause serious problems with our memory. Hypothyroidism and hypoglycemia can cause memory problems and distorted thinking.

Natural Therapy: Blood purification and a liver and kidney cleanse (toxins in the liver and kidneys are suspected as one cause of senility). Autointoxication is another cause of memory loss and senility. Cleansing the bowels with enemas, colonics or lower bowel formulas will help. A change of diet is necessary because often the elderly are not getting enough nutrients. They usually lack B-vitamins, vitamins E and C, and minerals. Calcium is lacking along with hydrochloric acid to help in assimilation of calcium. A hair analysis can determine heavy metal poisoning as well as a lack of vital minerals.

Foods to Heal: Most food intake should be raw or slow cooked to retain all nutrients. Seeds, whole grain, raw nuts, homemade yogurt. Brown rice, millet, buckwheat, wild rice. Eat plenty of fiber food. Use psyllium hulls to keep the colon clean. Fresh fruit and vegetable salads provide enzymes for assimilation. Organically-grown or soft-boiled eggs are good for memory retention. Foods high in nucleic acid containing DNA and RNA are salmon, sardines, oysters, soybeans, wheat germ and lentils. Bee pollen and spirulina also contain DNA and RNA.

Vitamins and Minerals: Lack of B-complex vitamins, especially B_1, are symptoms of a bad memory as well as lack of energy. B_{12} is involved with memory problems, depression and nervous system disorders. All the B vitamins work together. Vitamin A protects the immune system and is involved in keeping the mucous membranes, eyes, skin all healthy. Vitamin C with bioflavonoids help keep the arteries, and veins and capillaries healthy and clean. Vitamin E helps improve circulation to the brain. Multiminerals are vital for health. Calcium and magnesium, potassium, (use herbal formulas for proper assimilation of calcium), silicon, selenium (detoxifies heavy metals, drugs and her-

❖

bicides and pesticides), and zinc. Minerals help in detoxification of heavy metals.

Herbal Combinations: Bladder and kidney formulas, blood purifier (use red clover blend teas or formulas), chelation, digestion, glands, immune, liver and gallbladder and lower bowel formulas.

Single Herbs: Key herbs are dandelion (liver health), echinacea (cleans the lymphatics), garlic, gentian (keeps digestive system clean), ginkgo, ginseng, gotu kola (food for the brain), hawthorn (food for the heart and brain), hops (nourishes the nerves and brain), kelp, pau d'arco (great for blood and liver), prickly ash (circulation problems), red clover, skullcap (cleans the veins and protects nerves), suma. Other important herbs are alfalfa, black cohosh, black walnut (parasites and worms), capsicum (great for circulation), Oregon grape, yellow dock and yucca.

Supplements: Chlorophyll, green drinks and lecithin (contains choline which is important for healthy brain cells). Germanium and coenzyme Q_{10} are both important for circulation and brain function. Blue-green algae is good for clean veins so that pure blood can reach the brain.

Avoid: Avoid stress—it can lead to loss of nutrients to the brain cells. Avoid alcohol, caffeine, tobacco, fried foods and too much meat. Eat more fish. Avoid all products that contain aluminum or other heavy metals. Avoid a high-fat diet—it can clog up capillaries and arteries leading to the brain. Too much sugar and salt can contribute to the production of free radicals and loss of vital nutrients for brain health.

Dr. Paul Lofholm, consultant to the National Institute for Drug Abuse, makes us aware of another issue of senility: "Everyone knows that children need different dosages of drugs than adults. But it's only now being recognized that the adult dosages of most drugs should usually be cut in half for an older person because they absorb and excrete the drug at a much slower rate." Specialists often treat various diseases with drugs when they do not know what other doctors may have prescribed. A combination of medications can have serious adverse reactions. It has been estimated that a million Americans diagnosed as senile really suffer from a misuse of prescribed drugs, including large and harmful drug combinations. The dosages are much too high, and combinations of drugs from different doctors can produce symptoms diagnosed as senility. (From the National Institute For Drug Abuse.)

❖ SEXUALLY TRANSMITTED DISEASES (VENEREAL DISEASE)

Venereal disease is usually transmitted as a result of intimate contact through sexual intercourse. Syphilis and gonorrhea are the two most common types of sexually transmitted diseases. Chlamydia is another venereal disease that is occurring in epidemic proportions. It creates urinary tract problems in women and prostatic inflammation in men. It can also cause sterility in women.

These diseases are not going away, and medical treatment has not prevented the spread of these serious diseases by using antibiotics and other treatments. Other sexually transmitted diseases are chancroid, venerecum, granuloma, inguinal, genital herpes, and trichomoniasis.

Depending on the type of venereal disease the following symptoms may occur: painful urination, acute inflammation in the pelvic area, vaginal discharge, abnormal menstrual bleeding, brain damage, spinal cord damage, heart, liver, blood vessels or other vital organs of the body. Syphilis can cause insanity, paralysis, and death if not treated in time. If a pregnant woman has a venereal disease there is a pretty good chance her baby will be affected. This could mean birth defects, blindness, heart trouble, or even death.

Sexually transmitted diseases used to be treated with mercurial compounds; currently, they are usually treated with penicillin and other antibiotics. These diseases are acute so the body tries to clean and purify, but when they are suppressed by drugs the diseases are thrown deeper into the system to cause problems later. These are serious diseases and probably do need drugs, but after the treatment, effort must be made to clean the drugs from the system.

Natural Therapy: Germs and viruses will not attack a clean body. Work to keep the body clean both inside and out. Early treatment is necessary to prevent tissue damage. Afflicted persons should abstain from sexual intercourse and intimacy to prevent spreading the disease.

❖

Blood purification should be started along with lower bowel cleansing. If drugs are necessary, add acidophilus to prevent candida. Sitz baths will help ease pain and heal. Use herbs to help healing: pau d'arco, chaparral, red clover and black walnut in a sitz bath will help. Also use short fasts to clean the body of the impurities. There are also external goldenseal salves that will speed the healing.

Foods to Heal: Fruit will cleanse and purify the body. Eat cherries, grapes, plums, black currants, berries, papaya, lemons, limes, oranges and grapefruit. Eat the white of the citrus fruits because it is very healing. Vegetables are building, they contain a lot of minerals. Eat green peppers, parsley, broccoli, Brussels sprouts, cauliflower, red cabbage, chives, spinach, sprouts, and turnips. Protein is needed for tissue repair. Use almonds, sesame, chia, sunflower and pumpkin seeds. Millet and buckwheat contain protein and are easy to digest. Use a lot of fruit juices for healing and cleansing the body. Protein drinks will also help the healing process.

Vitamins and Minerals: High doses of vitamin A and C with bioflavonoids are very healing. Vitamins K and E will also help provide oxygen to the cells. Take a multimineral with extra silicon, selenium and zinc. Calcium, magnesium, manganese and potassium are also needed to help balance the pH factor in the body.

Herbal Combinations: Blood purifiers, candida, immune, infection formulas, lower bowels, parasites and worm formulas, stress and a bentonite cleanse will help.

Single Herbs: Key herbs are black walnut, burdock, chaparral, echinacea, garlic, gentian, goldenseal, kelp, oatstraw, pau d'arco, red clover, white oak and yellow dock. Other helpful herbs are alfalfa (contains vitamin K), buchu (cleans kidneys of impurities), capsicum, comfrey (tissue repair), fenugreek (helps clean the mucous membranes), hawthorn (protects the heart), horsetail (rich in silicon for healing), red raspberry, slippery elm (rich in protein for healing), uva ursi (cleans the kidneys), and yarrow.

Supplements: Acidophilus, chlorophyll, black walnut extract (use internally and externally), salmon oil, evening primrose oil, goldenseal extract, tea tree oil (external) and blue-green algae (helps purify the blood).

❖

Avoid: All sugar products, including candy, ice cream, cakes, pies, pastries. Also avoid all white flour products. They leach out the minerals that are necessary for healing. Avoid alcohol, tobacco, tea, coffee and chocolate.

❖ SHINGLES (HERPES ZOSTER)

Shingles is a disease that affects the nerve endings in the skin. It is caused by the same virus that causes chicken pox and it can occur in adults who had chicken pox as children. Some medical scientists feel that after a person is exposed to the chicken pox virus, it lies dormant in the body until it may be reactivated decades later in the form of shingles. Shingles is characterized by blister and crust formations as well as severe pain along the involved nerve. This could last for several weeks. The disease usually occurs on the chest and abdomen, but may occur on the face, around the eyes, on the forehead, neck and even the limbs and hands. The blisters will become crusty scabs and drop off. The elderly may suffer from attacks of shingles even after healing takes place. The pain may also continue for months after the symptoms disappear.

This is a virus that can lay dormant in the nerve ganglia and spinal cord for years until the immune system breaks down. This can be caused from vaccinations or from drugs used to suppress diseases. Shingles is an acute disease and so is a healing and cleansing of the body. When this disease is suppressed, it is pushed deeper into the system to cause even more serious problems. If this disease is treated naturally, it will only clean and heal the body.

Natural Therapy: With natural treatments of diseases you can start from the first appearance of the symptoms; you don't have to wait for days and numerous tests to find out what the disease is first. Fasting is the first law of nature to use with an acute disease. When eating during an acute disease, the body has to stop and use its energy to digest the food rather than eliminate toxins. Use blood purification along with lower bowel and kidney formulas. Use citrus juices, herbal teas and herbs to help nature do its job. The skin is called the third kidney. When the kidneys are plugged up, the skin has to take over. This is why the skin breaks out—it is trying to help the kidneys.

❖

Foods to Heal: Citrus juices are cleansing. Herbal teas will also help nature do its job: chamomile calms the nerves, alfalfa mint will help the stomach, red clover blend tea will help clean the blood, and pau d'arco will clean the blood and protect the liver. When healing has taken place with juices and fasting you can add vegetable broths, vegetables (steamed at first) and then raw salads and vegetables. Make a paste with aloe vera juice, black walnut, comfrey and powdered vitamin C to help the itching and speed healing.

Vitamins and Minerals: Massive doses of vitamin C will help speed the healing—some people have taken 10,000 mg a day to start with. Use vitamin C with bioflavonoids for better results. Vitamin C increases the activity of lymphocytes and improves the migration and mobility of leukocytes that help the immune system. Vitamin A will speed the healing of the rash. Calcium is necessary to assure assimilation of vitamins A, D and C. Vitamin E provides oxygen to the cells. B-complex vitamins are healing, and use extra B_{12} and B_1 until the symptoms disappear. A multimineral is very healing, with extra calcium and magnesium, potassium, manganese, silicon, selenium and zinc. A cream made with zinc will speed healing of the eruptions.

Herbal Combinations: Blood purifier, digestion, immune, lower bowels, kidney and bladder, nerves and stress formulas.

Single Herbs: Key herbs are aloe vera (internally and externally), black walnut (heals skin eruptions), blue vervain, comfrey, dandelion (helps the liver eliminate toxins), echinacea (helps the lymphatics to eliminate toxins), garlic (natural antibiotic), kelp, lady's slipper (excellent for the nerve endings), red clover, skullcap, wood betony and yellow dock. Other important herbs are the nervine herbs: black cohosh, hops, chamomile, passionflower and valerian.

Supplements: Use L-lysine with vitamin C, and cystine (detoxifies toxins). Good free-form amino acids are beneficial. Chlorophyll and rice bran syrup are helpful. Chinese essential oils (rub on blisters), essential fatty acids, salmon oil, evening primrose oil, safflower or olive oil (cold pressed only) and blue-green algae are also beneficial.

Avoid: Stop eating solid foods for the first three days to help nature cleanse. Avoid all sweet fruits, white sugar products, caffeine drinks, alcohol, and white flour products. Eliminate all white rice, pastries,

✤

sugar substitutes, and all junk food. They interfere with the cleansing and healing process. Avoid stress; take long walks in the fresh air and learn to have a positive attitude.

✤ SINUSITIS (SINUS INFECTION)

Sinusitis is an inflammation of one or more of the sinus cavities or passages located in the bones surrounding the eyes and nose. Acute sinusitis is usually caused by colds or bacterial and viral infections of the upper respiratory tract, nose or throat. Injury to the nasal bones and irritants such as fumes, air pollution, smoking and growths in the nose can cause chronic sinusitis.

An over-acid condition in the stomach will cause sinus infections. Infections are suspected if the mucus drainage is greenish or yellowish. Poor digestion of starch, sugar and dairy products will also cause a runny nose. Too much of one food and eating to excess can also cause sinus infections. Another thing that sometimes causes infections is allergies. If the drainage is clear and continues after a cold is gone, it usually means it is an allergy.

A typical sinus headache usually begins in the face under the cheekbones, often near the eyes. Sinusitis is usually caused by a cold, flu, measles, sore throat, infected tonsils, decayed teeth, enlarged and infected adenoids, cigarette smoke, and dusty air. Vitamin deficiencies can also be a cause. Vitamin A is essential for the health of the mucous membranes. Symptoms of sinusitis include facial pain, earache, headache, toothache, tenderness on the cheekbones, face and forehead.

In 1909 Dr. J. A. Stucky, M.D., published an article in the *Journal of the American Medical Association,* concerning intestinal autointoxication and conditions of the ears, nose and throat. He said, "Unsatisfactory results obtained after months of surgical and local treatment of some diseases of the ears, nose and throat have stimulated a more careful search for reasons why permanent relief was so rarely obtained. The question of intestinal autointoxication has at last come to the front where it belongs and has gained wide attention from the medical profession, both in Europe and America and the results and treatment of putrefaction and toxemia originating in the intestinal canal have become matters of great importance. We know that when the middle ear and nasal access sinus-

❖

es suffer from "air hunger" as a result of imperfect or obstructed drainage and ventilation, they do not function normally. Retained secretions become purulent (discharging pus), and lead to sepsis (poisoning caused by the absorption into the blood) and various functional disturbances: gastric, neurotic, circulatory and mental."

Natural Therapy: Sinusitis is an acute disease that needs to be treated naturally to prevent it from developing into a chronic condition. Blood purification, lower bowel cleansing, and a cleansing of the mucous membranes of the stomach are necessary for clearing up sinus infections. A change of diet that eliminates mucus-forming foods and introduces raw, nourishing whole foods will help. Fasting and using herbs will help dissolve hardened mucus that has accumulated in the sinuses for years. A tea made of goldenseal and fenugreek snuffed up the nose will help heal infections. Fenugreek will loosen the material and the goldenseal will heal. Fenugreek tea taken internally over a period of time will clean mucus from the body. Also use a hot water-vapor steam bath, using essential Chinese oils to make the sinuses feel better. With sinus problems a heavy breakfast in the morning is a mistake. In the morning the mucous linings and tubes in the sinus cavities are relaxed and in a cleansing state. Time and nutrients are needed for healing the mucous linings.

Foods to Heal: Juices (carrot and celery), green drinks, using pure apple juice or pineapple juice with parsley, watercress, carrot and celery tops, comfrey, chives and other greens are healing. For acute attacks, stop eating and use juices from lemons, limes, oranges or grapefruit. Pure water helps flush out toxins. Fruit juices are cleansing and vegetable juices are healing. Eat a lot of steamed vegetables and raw vegetable salads. Fresh fruit should be eaten in the morning, to help nature clean the mucous membranes.

Vitamins and Minerals: Take a lot of vitamin A during an acute attack (up to 10,000 I.U.) and vitamin B-complex with extra pantothenic acid. Vitamin C with bioflavonoids heal diseased mucous membranes. Multimineral tablets are also healing—calcium and magnesium, potassium, manganese, selenium, silicon, and zinc are needed.

Herbal Combinations: Allergy (usually contains ephedra for swelling), blood purifiers, candida, immune and infections formulas, lower bowels, digestion (for assimilation), lung and pain formulas.

Single Herbs: Key herbs are aloe vera (healing), ephedra, burdock, capsicum comfrey (repairs tissues), echinacea (for infections), fenugreek (dissolves mucus), garlic (antibiotic), ginger, goldenseal (antibiotic properties), lobelia, marshmallow, mullein, pau d'arco, red clover, rose hips, slippery elm (healing and provides protein for tissue repair), white oak and yellow dock.

Supplements: Bee pollen, chlorophyll, evening primrose oil, salmon oil, olive oil, blue-green algae.

Avoid: Mucus-forming foods such as milk, cheese, meat, too many starches, sugar, salt, and pastries. Do not take sinus medications—they stop the cleansing process.

❖ SKIN PROBLEMS (ECZEMA, DERMATITIS, PSORIASIS)

The skin has a vital function in eliminating toxins, gases, pollution and vapor from the system. Two quarts of these toxins are released every day if the pores are clean and free from the buildup of dead cells. If the skin is closed because of dead cell buildup, these toxins are thrown back into the body for the other organs of elimination to take over.

When the body has enough energy and vitality and the blood is clean, the channels of elimination will take care of the toxins that are not eliminated through the skin. But if the body is overloaded with waste and toxic material, and if the bowels and kidneys are already weakened through continued over-work and over-stimulation, nature causes an acute disease to manifest itself. In effect, the body is attempting a natural elimination to get rid of the waste and poisons causing low vitality in the body.

When the body is overloaded with toxins and then exposed to drafts, cold, and wet weather, the toxic matter is thrown into the circulation. When the skin is chilled, the pores close causing and it causes the blood to recede into the internal organs. As a result the elimination of poisonous gases, vapors and toxins are suppressed. If the other normal channels of elimination are also shut down then the toxins are thrown into the mucous linings and cause irritation to the nasal passages, throat, bronchi, stomach, lungs or the genito-urinary organs. This produces the symptoms of inflammation, infections, catarrhal elimination, sneezing, coughs, runny nose, diarrhea, leucorrhea, etc.

Skin diseases are a sign of toxic irritation. A film of dirt and pollution accumulates daily on the surface of the skin. When the body is overloaded with mucus and fat deposits, the kidney, liver and digestive organs cannot process and eliminate fast enough and therefore the body expels through the skin. When the skin is not properly cleansed, the dead cells, rancid oil, perspiration, wastes and bacteria accumulate and cause blackheads, pimples and whiteheads.

Natural Therapy: Blood purification and lower bowel cleansing. The liver and kidneys need to be cleaned of impurities. Skin brushing will help keep the skin clean and allow the pores to eliminate excess toxins. Juice fasting will help keep the blood clean. Exercise is beneficial for lymphatic cleansing, and the elimination of toxins. Besides brushing, the skin needs massage, fresh air, exercise, sunlight, and hot and cold showers.

Foods to Heal: Carrots and carrot juice. Apricots, kale, mustard, spinach, collard greens, parsley, turnip greens, mustard greens, cabbage, chives, watercress, sweet red pepper and green peppers and winter squash are all high in vitamin A. Fruit is healing and steamed vegetables are high in minerals. Eat lots of green salads. Brown rice (thermos cooked) will retain nutrients for healing the skin. Millet is easily assimilated.

Vitamins and Minerals: Vitamin A is needed for skin health. B-complex with extra B_2, B_6 and niacin is helpful. Vitamin D works with vitamin A for skin health. Vitamin E used internally and externally will help maintain a healthy skin. Multiminerals are essential for proper skin function. Silicon (heals skin irritations), selenium and zinc are also involved in skin healing. Potassium, manganese, calcium and magnesium are also necessary.

Herbal Combinations: Allergy blood purifiers, bone (rich in silicon and other minerals), digestion, hair and skin formulas, immune, liver and gallbladder, lower bowels, nerve, potassium and stress combinations.

Single Herbs: Key herbs are alfalfa (rich in vitamin A and minerals), aloe vera, burdock, comfrey (heals and builds cells), dandelion, goldenseal, horsetail, oatstraw, queen of the meadow, red clover, skullcap and yellow dock (rich in iron). Other important herbs are buchu (cleans kidneys), capsicum, chaparral (cleans blood and eliminates toxins), cornsilk (kidney and bladder cleanser), echinacea, fenugreek, gotu kola, hawthorn, hops, ho-shou-wu, lady's slipper, lobelia, mistletoe, pau d'arco, wood betony and wormwood.

Supplements: Aloe vera juice (external and internal), evening primrose oil, salmon oil, lecithin, black ointment (external for healing), Chinese essential oils, chlorophyll, redmond clay (external), tea tree oil (external).

Avoid: High-fat and high-meat diet. Eliminate alcohol, tobacco and caffeine drinks. Reduce sugar and white flour products. Don't use birth control pills. Some drugs cause skin problems. Avoid salt, rancid oils, soft drinks, chocolate, potato chips and all junk food.

✢ STRESS

Everyone is plagued with stress. It should not be considered all bad as long as we are capable of handling situations we need to face. Stress can be beneficial and can challenge and motivate us to accomplish the seemingly impossible task. The way we choose to deal with stress is the key to coping with it. If not controlled properly, stress can become "distress." Stressful situations can build up time and take a toll on our physical and emotional health. We need to strengthen our bodies so we can withstand any stress we need to. It is important to learn to avoid stress we cannot handle and to handle stress we cannot avoid. Some ways to do this are nutritionally building our nerves, fortifying our immune system, and learning to relax and exercise.

Stress can accumulate in the body and eventually cause a breakdown of the adrenal glands. This will cause exhaustion and a complete weakening of the emotional and physical body. It may take twenty years to accomplish this, but it will happen if long-term stress is allowed to continue. It could be a high-pressure job, a bad marriage, unresolved financial problems, loneliness or a death in the family. It isn't the situation you are in, it's how you cope with your life situations.

When the body is completely burned out because of nutrient lack, stress can control life's situation. The body, especially the nerves, have to be nourished and fed. Sugar is one of the worst things you can put in

✧

the body that will wear it down and cause exhaustion. Sugar depletes nutrients from the system. Yet we use sugar to give us a lift, only to have the adrenals eventually burn out. Symptoms of adrenal exhaustion are chronic fatigue, irritability, health problems, anxiety, depression, low stress tolerance, the feeling of being unable to cope or stay in touch with reality, nervous exhaustion, insomnia, difficulty in relaxing, and panic attacks.

Natural Therapy: Relaxation therapy is an art to learn. It is possible for anyone to use and benefit from it. Blood purification, and lower bowel cleansing. This will keep the blood clean so that toxins cannot travel to the brain and nerves and cause stress. A nutritional diet is necessary. A change of diet is the first step in conquering stress.

Foods to Heal: The following foods are rich in vitamin A, calcium, and vitamin C: carrots and carrot juice, yams, kale, parsley, turnip greens, collard greens, swiss chard, watercress, red and green peppers, winter squash, egg yolk, endive, persimmons, apricots, broccoli, leaf lettuce, peaches, cherries, strawberries, oranges, grapefruit, cantaloupe, green onions, limes, tangerines, tomatoes and raspberries. Foods high in magnesium and other essential minerals are blackstrap molasses, sunflower seeds, whole grains, almonds, soybeans, pecans, hazelnuts, oats, brown rice, millet, white and red beans, wild rice, rye, beet greens, lentils, dried figs, lima beans, apricots, dried dates, peaches, okra and parsley.

Vitamins and Minerals: Vitamin A promotes growth and repair of body tissues. It is used up quickly when a person is under stress. B-vitamins are known as the "stress vitamins." They fortify the nervous system. Many people will not take B-vitamins because they say the vitamins makes them sick. The reason is that the liver is adjusting to having nutrients and needs time to adjust to good nutrition. The liver is also filtering out toxins. Folic acid aids in the assimilation of pantothenic acid. PABA is needed to aid in the production of pantothenic acid. Vitamin C stimulates adrenal function and protects vitamin E, calcium, hormones, and enzymes from destruction. Vitamin E protects the glands when under stress. Take a multimineral supplement with extra calcium for the nerves. Potassium aids in insomnia; magnesium

❖

calms the nerves. Selenium is good for immune protection and zinc nourishes the thymus gland, which can be destroyed from stress.

Herbal Combinations: Blood purifier, immune, lower bowel, nerve and stress formulas.

Single Herbs: Key herbs are alfalfa, chamomile, ginkgo (strengthens the brain), gotu kola (brain food), hops, kelp, lady's slipper, licorice, lobelia, mistletoe, mullein, passionflower, pau d'arco, rose hips (rich in B-vitamins), skullcap (improves nerves), suma (builds immunity), valerian, and wood betony.

Supplements: Bee pollen, evening primrose oil, salmon oil, lecithin (feeds the nerves), blue-green algae, acidophilus and chlorophyll (cleans the blood).

Avoid: Tranquilizers. They eventually cause more stress than they alleviate. Eliminate all drugs be cause they put stress on the body. Over-the-counter drugs deplete the body of nutrients that protect against stress. Avoid white sugar products, white flour products, rancid oils, fried foods. Be aware that alcohol, tobacco and caffeine will deplete the body and cause stress.

❖ STROKES

A stroke is a loss of functioning brain tissue, either temporary or permanent. There are two kinds of strokes. One type is cerebral hemorrhage, caused by a weak place in a blood vessel in the brain giving way. Such a hemorrhage is most likely to happen to those with high blood pressure. It can also happen to those with clogged and weak arteries. The second kind of stroke is cerebral thrombosis, due to a clot or other blockage in a blood vessel in the brain. Some health-oriented doctors who have treated thousands of people suffering from stroke feel that most strokes can be prevented.

A mild attack can cause temporary confusion and light headedness, difficulty in speaking clearly, weakness on one side of the body, vision dimness and confusion, severe speech difficulties, and/or sudden or gradual loss or blurring of consciousness. Amnesia can also occur, but is often not permanent. A coma can result for short or long periods.

Some early warnings of stroke—which may only last for a few moments—include one or more of the following: fainting, stumbling, numbness or paralysis of the fingers of one hand, blurring of vision, seeing bright lights, loss of speech or memory. It is much wiser and less expensive to start improving health in order to prevent this disease.

A poisoned blood stream sets the stage for a possible stroke. Poisoned blood flows through thousands of miles of arteries, veins, and capillaries. The walls of the arteries consist of cells which are subject to the same injury from toxins as the cells in the kidneys. The kidneys degenerate at the same time the arteries do and from the same causes. When the walls thicken and harden, this causes degeneration. As they harden they become more brittle and more easily burst under pressure. Pressure increases as the hole through the arteries grows smaller. As the walls become more brittle, extra pressure causes a blood vessel to rupture, which causes a stroke. The brain cells rely on oxygen-rich blood for nourishment. If they don't receive this nourishment, the brain cells die.

Natural Therapy: Blood purification, stimulation therapy, lower bowel cleansing. A natural oral chelation will clean the entire system and help the blood flow freely. It will improve circulation so that proper nutrition and oxygen can reach the brain. Short fasting and a change of diet will also help to clean the arteries. High blood pressure severely strains the arteries, and if the arteries have cholesterol plaques, it can set the body up for a stroke. Stress is a big contributor of strokes, yet stress is hard to determine. A person isn't usually aware they are under stress. Someone who is always angry or hateful has an extra excretion of hormones and acids, raising blood pressure and contributing to strokes or heart disease.

Foods to Heal: High-fiber foods such as whole grains (oats, wheat, barley, millet, buckwheat) contain rutin which strengthens the veins. Brown rice, wild rice, beans, nuts, and seeds contain nutrients for capillary health. Vegetables are rich in minerals and low in calories. Potatoes, carrots, celery, cauliflower, cabbage, beets, onions, cucumbers, and green peppers are nutritious. Use leaf lettuce, tomatoes, greens, string beans, snow peas, and sweet potatoes. Onions, garlic, scallions, ginger and cayenne pepper have anticlotting effects.

Vitamins and Minerals: Vitamins A and E are antioxidants, bringing more oxygen to the blood and acting as free radical scavengers.

❖

Vitamin E is essential for supplying oxygen to the heart muscles. Vitamin C with bioflavonoids protects the capillaries and cleans and strengthens the veins. The B-complex vitamins improves overall good health. They improve liver function, feed the nerves and brain, and help clean and feed the veins. Minerals are essential for pure blood and to keep the body's chemistry in balance. Iron is essential to supply oxygen to the cells. Selenium and zinc protect the immune system. Silicon helps the body utilize calcium and prevent it from adhering to the veins. Potassium is necessary for a healthy heart. Calcium and magnesium are needed for nerves and brain.

Herbal Combinations: Heart and blood pressure formulas, glands, nerves, bone, chelation, digestion, potassium.

Single Herbs: Key herbs are capsicum (cleans veins, strengthens the walls of the arteries), bugleweed (alleviates pain in heart), burdock, butcher's broom (improves circulation), ephedra, garlic, ginkgo (improves mental clarity), gotu kola (feeds the brain), hawthorn, hops, horsetail, kelp, passionflower, parsley, pau d'arco, psyllium, rose hips, saffron, skullcap and valerian. Other important herbs are alfalfa (rich in minerals), black cohosh (for slow pulse rate), blessed thistle, dandelion, ginseng, lily of the valley, lobelia and yellow dock.

Supplements: Chlorophyll (rebuilds heart), lecithin (prevents fatty deposits), flaxseed, evening primrose oil, salmon oil, glucomannan, rice bran syrup, coenzyme Q_{10}, germanium.

Avoid: Constipation—it throws toxins into the bloodstream which weaken the blood vessels. Also avoid smoking, alcohol and drugs of all kinds. Chlorinated water can weaken the veins. High-fat and meat diets weaken the veins. Avoid too many dairy products. Try to eliminate stress by changing to a more relaxing lifestyle.

❖ TICKS, LICE, BED BUGS, FLEAS (LYME DISEASE, ROCKY MOUNTAIN SPOTTED FEVER)

Ticks, lice, bed bugs and fleas cannot live in a clean body. Not everyone is infested with them, but those whose internal and external conditions supply the little varmints with food to support their life can suffer. For this reason it is important that the body and blood are cleaned and purified.

Head lice are most often found on the scalp and hair, behind the ears and at the back of the neck. The tiny nits (eggs) are laid at the base of a hair shaft and the attached egg moves away from the scalp as the hair grow. Itching is one symptom, and sometimes you can actually see the lice and eggs, which may look like dandruff.

Crab lice are transmitted mainly by sexual contact and are found in the genital areas. They can also be transmitted by using a toilet seat where infestation is present. Itching is a symptom as well as the appearance of tiny black dots clinging to the base of the hairs. The lice can spread to the eyelashes, beard, or hair on the chest.

Many people feel that lice are a sign of uncleanliness. They are, but it does not mean you live in filth. It means that the body has either inherited weakness or has acquired toxins that contribute to these infestations. White sugar in the body contributes to these bugs.

Tick bites can cause Rocky Mountain spotted fever and Lyme disease. An epidemic of these ticks have been seen in some areas. Children should be inspected after playing outside in wooded, brushy areas, especially in late spring and summer. Prevention is the best weapon. Ticks can be seen before they do their dangerous job. It takes several minutes for them to drill into the skin so inspecting yourselves and your children is the best prevention.

Natural Therapy: Blood purifying and lower bowel cleansing to prevent toxins from staying in the blood. All bugs and parasites live on the toxins that have accumulated in the body from what we call autointoxication. Dr. Henry Lindlahr used diet, cold water treatment and a comb to get rid of lice and other bugs. He said that treating them with antiseptics and strong drugs would only push them further into the body, especially in the head area, and cause headaches, dizziness, loss of memory, deafness and weak eyesight. To remove ticks that have imbedded into the body, first pour on alcohol or olive oil to smother the tick and than carefully twist the tick with a pair of tweezers and gently pull. If the head is left in it could cause infections. With body lice, bed bugs, and any similar bug, the clothing should be sterilized. They live only on the body when they want to feed. Soak combs and brushes in Lysol with hot water for about thirty minutes. Freezing

❖

will also kill bugs. A solution of vinegar, lemon juice and olive oil can be applied at night for a couple of hours. Try to use natural methods to prevent pushing them further in the body for problems later on. For the hair and other areas make a solution of goldenseal, black walnut and aloe vera juice. Put it on the area for about an hour, then shampoo or wipe off.

Foods to Heal: Fruit is cleansing for the body. Use organic fruit if possible. Bugs cannot live in a clean body. Wheat grass juice is very beneficial to cleanse and nourish the blood. Green drinks using pure apple juice or pineapple juice with sprouts, spinach, comfrey, and parsley or any green leafy vegetables are excellent. Sulphur vegetables will help kill the eggs and bugs. They are horseradish, kale, cabbage, Brussels sprouts, cauliflower, chervil and watercress. Other foods high in sulphur are cranberries, turnips, spinach, savoy cabbage, red cabbage, parsnip, leek, onions, garlic, kohlrabi, radishes, okra, swiss chard and chives. Put ground pumpkin seeds on your food every day.

Vitamins and Minerals: A clean body, both inside and out, is essential. Vitamins and minerals help keep the body clean. Vitamin A heals the mucous membranes and protects the immune system. B-complex vitamins protect the nerves. Vitamin C with bioflavonoids helps protect the cells and immune system. Vitamin E supplies oxygen to the cells. Multiminerals are vital. Calcium and magnesium, sulphur, selenium, and zinc protect the body. Selenium, vitamin A, and vitamin E are antioxidants and free radical scavengers that protects the cells.

Herbal Combinations: Blood purifiers, digestion, immune, liver, lower bowel formulas, parasites formulas and potassium.

Single Herbs: Key herbs are black walnut (kills parasites and worms), burdock (cleans blood), chaparral (purifies blood), garlic, goldenseal, horsetail, kelp, pau d'arco, psyllium, red clover, senna, wormwood and yellow dock. Other beneficial herbs are alfalfa, aloe vera, buchu, cornsilk, echinacea, hops, gotu kola, lobelia, papaya, parsley, peppermint, St. John's wort, uva ursi, wood betony and yarrow.

Supplements: Chlorophyll, bentonite, diatomaceous earth, garlic extract, glucomannan, spirulina.

Avoid: All junk food, fried food, white sugar and white flour products. Eliminate pastries, cookies, candy and ice cream. Avoid meat, even chicken can harbor bugs. Use a natural insect repellent to avoid ticks and other bugs.

❖ TONSILLITIS AND STREP THROAT

Tonsillitis does not necessarily mean there is a strep infection. But tonsillitis, sore throat, swollen glands in the neck, sinusitis, and middle ear infections could mean a streptococcus infection is present. The strep germ can do much harm and indirectly cause rheumatic fever and nephritis (kidney disease).

When a child does not seem to be recovering from a cold, sore throat or bronchial infection, or if a fever develops when a cold seems to be subsiding, this may suggest a potential serious complication. Also, if fever, headaches and vomiting continue and the throat becomes so sore that it is hard to swallow, a health doctor should be consulted.

The tonsils are one of the body's protections against airborne bacteria entering the system through the mouth and nose. These work with the lymphatic system to fight infections. When the tonsils become inflamed, it is nature's way of telling you to clean out the body. When sore throats are constantly irritated with drugs (which suppress the acute disease), overeating, and lack of rest, the mucus the body is trying to eliminate is thrown back into the system to cause a worse problem next time. If the tonsils continue to become inflamed, scar tissue will eventually accumulate and prevent the tonsils from doing what nature intended. If you have lost both your tonsils and appendix through surgery, an extra burden is put on the lymphatics.

Natural Therapy: Blood purification and lower bowel cleansing are needed. A three-day juice fast will help. Use citrus juices, herbal teas, herbal extracts, chiropractic, foot reflexology and massage therapy for improved circulation. If you eat during the cleansing process (acute diseases are nature's way of cleansing and healing the body), the body has to stop and digest food, which puts toxins further into the body to emerge as a chronic disease later. Bed rest and relaxation are necessary for the body to heal itself. Enemas, colonics or herbal bowel cleansers will speed the healing process. This will bring the fever down in a natural way.

Foods to Heal: Citrus juices, oranges, lemons, limes and grapefruit will cleanse the lymphatics. Herbal teas help nature clean and eliminate the toxins. Pure water and herbal teas flush out the toxins that cells release into the stomach.

Vitamins and Minerals: Vitamin A needs to be taken in high amounts at first. Vitamin C with bioflavonoids will heal and flush out the toxins. Vitamin B-complex is needed to rebuild after an acute disease has passed. Take a multimineral with extra calcium and magnesium (in herbal form), potassium, selenium, silicon and zinc.

Herbal Combinations: Blood purifier, allergy formulas, cold and flu formulas, infection, lower bowel, nerve and potassium formulas.

Single Herbs: Key herbs are alfalfa and mint tea, aloe vera (laxative and attracts toxins to be eliminated), fenugreek and comfrey together (break up mucus), echinacea (a special herb to help clean the lymphatics), ginger (settles stomach), goldenseal (a strong antibiotic), kelp (will clean and nourish), lobelia (the greatest healer of the stomach which is the center of disease), marshmallow (healing to the mucous membranes), passionflower, hops, skullcap (all nervine herbs will relax the body for nature to heal), red raspberry (in tea form for fast assimilation), pau d'arco (protects the liver and cleans the blood), rose hips (rich in vitamin C and B-complex vitamins) and slippery elm (for coughs and healing the throat and stomach).

Supplements: Green drinks, chlorophyll, lemon-lime drinks mixed with herbal extracts, rice bran syrup, essential fatty acids, evening primrose oil, salmon oil and Chinese essential oils (rub on throat and neck to help pain).

Avoid: Stop eating during an acute disease. Avoid caffeine, alcohol, tobacco, and over-the-counter drugs. They will only suppress elimination. Avoid sugar and white flour products.

❖ ULCERS

Ulcers are one of the plagues of modern-day living. It has been well established that emotional stress and anxiety are two of the main causes of gastric ulcers. The pit of the stomach is often used as a sounding board for our emotions. Nine out of ten people who acquire ulcers get them through worrying over existing (or non-existing) problems in life.

It seems that in order to prevent gastric ulcers there is a need to find ways to handle life's problems that will not affect the stomach. There has to be a way to combat tensions that will prevent the stomach from suffering.

Autointoxication and constipation are other causes of ulcers. When the lower colon is clogged it delays the passage of food from the system. Fermentation and acid conditions which irritate the stomach wall will result. During acute disease the cells eliminate toxins into the stomach to be removed from the body through the colon. When diseases are suppressed with drugs or eating, it stops the cleansing and the stomach becomes irritated. When this is done, it often weakens the stomach muscles.

An ulcer simply means an open sore. Peptic ulcers indicate that the sore is in the stomach or the duodenum, the first part of the intestines which connect with the stomach. They are associated with the presence of an excessive amount of acid gastric juice. Worry and anxiety increase the secretion of the stomach. You should never eat when you are worried or feel anxious.

The most common symptom of an ulcer is a burning sensation or discomfort in the upper abdomen, usually felt about two or three hours after meals or in the middle of the night. Nausea and vomiting may occur. Sometimes an ulcer will cause bleeding, and a slow seeping of blood may cause anemia.

Natural Therapy: Tranquilization therapy using nervine herbs to strengthen the nervous system. The stomach feels every emotion you have and needs to be healed. With stomach ulcers, a person's vitality and strength are weakened, so they need to repair and heal. If constipation is the problem, enemas and juice fasts can help. Freshly squeezed cabbage juice will heal ulcers. Aloe vera juice is also healing as it inhibits the secretion of hydrochloric acid. Proper chewing is essential as is proper food combining to give the stomach time for healing. Doctors used to recommend bland diets but now find that they are not beneficial because they contain no nourishment.

Foods to Heal: Slippery elm is an herb that is considered a food. It will heal ulcers and also provide protein and nourishment. Potatoes are

healing; they have an alkaline reaction and help neutralize acid production. Bake them at 500 degrees to change them from a starch to
glucose. Well-chewed almonds will help and do not cause an over-
production of acid. Almond milk helps to neutralize excess acid in the
stomach. Carrots and carrot juice will heal and are very high in calcium and vitamin A. millet, brown rice, buckwheat and yellow corn
meal will heal, but need to be cooked slowly in a thermos to retain
enzymes. Rejuvelac is a healthy enzyme drink. It acts as a protection
against harmful organisms in the intestinal tract. It is rich in protein,
carbohydrates, B-complex vitamins and vitamins E and K. (K protects against bleeding).

Barley helps to rebuild the lining of the stomach and soothes
ulcers with its rich content of B_1 and B_2, and bioflavonoids. Cook
slowly in a thermos to retain the B-vitamins. Okra powder acts as a
demulcent to stop inflammation. Eat papaya often. It contains
enzymes to improve digestion and is very healing to the stomach lining. Persimmon, an energy food, also heals and soothes the mucous
membranes of the stomach. Sprouts contain live enzymes, protein,
vitamins and minerals. Sweet potatoes are soothing and nourishing.
Whey powder contains natural sodium that is healing to ulcers.

Vitamins and Minerals: Vitamin A protects the stomach acid from irritation. Vitamins A and E together protect against ulcers developing
as well as heal. Vitamin C with bioflavonoids will heal ulcers. Vitamin
E will also heal scar tissues. (Remember all sores cause scar tissue to
form). Minerals are important in healing ulcers. Iron builds rich
blood and helps restore vitality. Vitamin K prevents bleeding.
Calcium and magnesium heal the nerves and help in ulcers.
Potassium helps balance excess acid. Selenium, silicon and zinc help
heal ulcers.

Herbal Combinations: Blood purifiers, bone (rich in minerals), comfrey
and pepsin, digestion, lower bowels, nerve and ulcer formulas.

Single Herbs: Key herbs are alfalfa (rich in minerals and vitamins, especially K), aloe vera, capsicum, comfrey, fenugreek, garlic, goldenseal
(very healing for the digestive system), hops (for the nerves), kelp,
lady's slipper, lobelia, oatstraw, pau d'arco, psyllium, skullcap, slippery elm and white oak. Other important herbs are black walnut,

❖

burdock, dandelion, echinacea, ginger, hawthorn, myrrh, watercress and yellow dock (rich in iron).

Supplements: Aloe vera juice, liquid chlorophyll, glucomannan, evening primrose oil, salmon oil and blue-green algae. Bee pollen helps heal the digestive system. Flaxseed tea coats the digestive tract and protects the sores. (Simmer two tablespoons in a pint of water for about three or four minutes.) Propolis heals ulcers and contains antibiotic properties.

Avoid: Heated vegetable oil may cause ulcers. Don't eat when under stress. Antacids can upset the metabolic balance of the body. Cimetidine is widely prescribed for ulcer pain but does nothing to cure the ulcers. It could cause cancer and even sterility. Aspirin can cause bleeding and ulcers. Smoking inhibits pancreatic bicarbonate secretion and can cause ulcers. Food stagnation can cause ulcers. Avoid white sugar and flour; they stimulate acid production.

BIBLIOGRAPHY

Austin, Phylis, Agatha Thrash, M.D. and Calvin Thrash, M.D., M.P.H., *Natural Healthcare For Your Child*, 1990. Published by Family Health Publication, Sunfield, Mich.

Balch, James F., M.D. and Balch, Phyllis A. C.N.C., 1990. Published by Avery Publishing Group, Inc., Garden City Park, New York.

Baroody, Theodore A., Jr., M.A., D.C., 1987. Published by OMNI Learning Institute, Asheville, N.C.

Cayetano, H.J.M., Building Vital Health, 1988. Published by The Eastern Publishing Association, Manila.

Douglass, William Campbell, M.D. Aids The End of Civilization, 1989. Published by Valet Publishers, Clayton, Georgia.

Galland, Leo, M.D., with Dian Dincin Buchaman, Ph.D. Superimmunity for Kids. 1988. Published by Delta Book, New York, N.Y.

Hoffman, David, The Holistic Herbal, 1983. Published by The Findhorn Press, Scotland.

James, Walene, Immunization The Reality Behind The Myth, 1988. Published by Gergen & Gravey Publishers, Inc., Massachusetts.

Fox, William, M.D., Family Botanic Guide or Every Man His Own Doctor, 1904.

Lindlahr, Henry, M.D., Natural Therapeutics, Vol. 1, 2 and 6. Philosophy of Natural Therapeutics, 1918. Practice of Natural Therapeutics, 1919. Iridiagnosis and other Diagnostic Methods, 1922.

Mudd, Chris, Cholesterol and Your Health, The Great American Rip Off. Published by American Lite Co., Oklahoma City, OK.

Pierce, R.V., M.D., The Peoples Common Sense Medical Adviser, 1895.

Roberts, Frank, Modern Herbalism for Digestive Disorders, 1978. Published by Thorsons Publishing Limited, England.

Lust, John, N.D. and Michael Tierra, C.A., O.M.D. The Natural Remedy Bible. Published by Pocket Book, Simon and Schuster, 1990.

Lad, Dr. Vasant and Frawley, David, The Yoga of Herbs, 1986. Published by Lotus Press, Santa Fe, New Mexico.

LePore, Donald, N.D., The Ultimate Healing System, 1985. Published by Woodland Books, Provo, Utah.

Muramoto, Noboru, Natural Immunity, Insights on Diet and Aids. 1988. Published by George Ohsawa Macrobiotic Foundation, Oroville, California.

Stevens, Dr. John, Medical Reform or Physiology and Botanic Practice, London, 1847.

Santilli, Humbart, B.S., M.H. Natural Healing with Herbs, 1984. Published by Hohm Press, Prescott Valley, AZ.

Scott, Julian, Ph.D. Natural Medicine for Children, 1990. Published by Avon Books,

❖

New York, N.Y.

Stone, Dr. Randolph, D.O., D.C., 1985. Published by CRCS Published, Sebastopol, California.

Tenney, Louise M.H. Today's Herbal Health, Today's Healthy Eating, Modern Day Plagues and Health Handbook. Published by Woodland Books, Provo, Utah.

Thomson, Samuel, 1835. New Guide To Health or Botanic Family Physician.

Tierra, Michael, C.A., N.D., The Way of Herbs, 1980. Published by Unity Press, Santa Cruz, California. Planetary Herbology, 1988. Published by Lotus Press, Santa Fe, New Mexico.

Theiss, Barbara and Peter, The Family Herbal, 1989. Published by Healing Arts Press, Rochester, Vermont.

Truss, C. Orian, M.D. The Missing Diagnosis, 1983. Published by The Missing Diagnosis, Inc., Birmingham, Alabama.

Weiss, Rudolf, Fritz, M.D., Herbal Medicine, 1988. Distributed by Medicina Biologica, Portland, Oregon.

Welles, William F., D.C., The Shocking Truth About Cholesterol, 1990. Published by William F. Welles, D.C.

Willard, Terry, Ph.D., Helping Yourself with Natural Remedies, 1951. Published by CRCS Publications, Reno, Nevada.

INDEX

❖

❖

❖

❖

❖

❖

❖

❖

❖

❖